The Fear of Table Sugar

Understanding the Myths and Realities of Sugar Consumption

Brenda F. Dozier

Gratitude

Dear Reader,

Thank you for purchasing The Fear of Table Sugar: Understanding the Myths and Realities of Sugar Consumption. Your choice to invest in this book is a testimonial to your commitment to getting a deeper understanding of the frequently misunderstood topic of sugar. It is readers like you who motivate us to continue our pursuit of clarity and truth in a world flooded with information.

Your willingness to explore the complexity of sugar consumption demonstrates a dedication to personal health and well-being. We are honored to be a part of your journey toward making informed food choices and knowing the science behind the sweet substance that has become a staple in our lives.

We know that your time is valuable, and we appreciate that you have chosen to spend it with us. Our objective is to present you with a comprehensive, engaging, and instructive read that will empower you with the information to navigate the often-perplexing terrain of nutrition.

Writing this book has been a labor of love, inspired by the desire to distinguish fact from fantasy and present you with practical knowledge that you can implement in your daily life. We hope that the information offered within these pages will not only educate but also motivate you to make decisions that correspond with your health goals.

Your support means the world to us. It is through your readership that we can share our love for health and nutrition with a wider audience. If this book has sparked questions, provided answers, or motivated you to reevaluate your relationship with sugar, then our mission has been fulfilled.

Thank you once again for your trust and for allowing us to be a part of your health journey. We wish you success in your endeavors to lead a healthier, more informed life.

With sincere gratitude,

[Brenda F. Dozier]

Table of Contents

Introduction

Welcome to "The Fear of Table Sugar: Understanding the Myths and Realities of Sugar Consumption." By reading this book, you will gain a better understanding of table sugar, which is one of the most contentious and misunderstood components of our diet. As you go through this book, you will uncover the truths that have been concealed beneath the veil of fear that has surrounded sugar for many years.

Sugar has played a significant role throughout human history, with its presence integrated into every aspect of our civilizations, rituals, and everyday lives. However, in recent years, it has begun to play the role of the antagonist in the narrative of our health. There are several worrying myths that you may have heard, such as "Sugar is as addictive as cocaine," "It is the root cause of obesity and diabetes," and "Feeding your child sugar is comparable to poisoning them." Fear and anxiety are triggered as a result of these comments, which frequently result in significant dietary adjustments that may not be supported by solid scientific evidence. It is the purpose of this book to create clarity by providing a balanced perspective that can cut through the noise.

There is a fork in the path for our society. On the one hand, we are inundated with marketing messages from the food business, which is always trying to entice us with sugary delicacies at this exact moment. On the other hand, we are flooded with dire warnings from health professionals and media outlets, pushing us to remove sugar. Where does the truth lie? How do we navigate these contradicting signals to make educated choices for ourselves and our families? This book is designed to guide you through this maze with evidence-based insights and practical recommendations.

Imagine a world where you could eat your favorite delicacies without a rising cloud of shame and misunderstanding. A world where you understand the true role of sugar in your diet, its possible hazards, and its place in a balanced lifestyle. This book attempts to empower you with knowledge, refuting the myths and revealing the facts about sugar consumption. We'll cover the science, the history, and the cultural significance of sugar, equipping you with the tools to make informed decisions for yourself and your family.

Is sugar truly the main factor behind the obesity epidemic? Does it directly cause diabetes, or are there more subtle elements at play? These questions and more will be explored extensively.

But this book doesn't stop at refuting falsehoods. It empowers you with the information to manage your sugar intake without falling victim to fear-mongering. You will learn how to spot hidden sugars in your food, make healthier choices, and enjoy your meals without guilt. Whether you are a parent concerned about your child's food, someone suffering from weight management, or simply an inquisitive reader wanting to make sense of contradicting information, this book is for you.

We live in an age where information is available but not necessarily reliable. "The Fear of Table Sugar" tries to cut through disinformation and offer you the tools to make balanced, informed decisions about your diet. By the end of this book, you will have a thorough grasp of what sugar is, how it affects your body, and how you can enjoy it in moderation without compromising your health.

Join us on this enlightening journey. Let's replace fear with information, misconceptions with facts, and confusion with clarity. This book is not just about understanding sugar; it's about regaining control over your health and choosing decisions that are best for you. Dig in, and uncover the truth about table sugar. Your journey to informed and empowered eating starts here.

Hook: A Personal Anecdote or Startling Fact About Sugar Consumption

It was a sunny summer afternoon when I found myself in a small, lively café in New York City. I observed as a mother offered her toddler a brilliantly colored lollipop. The child's eyes lit up with sheer excitement, an emotion that seemed nearly universal. Across the room, a young woman stirred three packets of sugar into her iced coffee, relishing the flavor with a happy sigh. Moments later, a middle-aged man at the next table pulled out a granola bar, a so-called "healthy" snack that had nearly as much sugar as a candy bar. These snapshots of daily life can appear banal, yet they reflect a deeper truth about our collective connection with sugar. It is omnipresent, enmeshed in our rituals and habits, yet often ingested without a second thought about its repercussions.

Consider this astonishing fact: the average American consumes around 17 teaspoons of added sugar per day, significantly above the recommended maximum of 6 teaspoons for women and 9 teaspoons for men stated by the American Heart Association. This high intake has been linked to many health concerns, from obesity and diabetes to heart disease and teeth damage. Despite these well-documented hazards, sugar intake continues to climb, driven by the potent combination of human desires and the food industry's continuous push to add sugar to an ever-expanding assortment of products.

The Sweet Paradox: Discuss the Love-Hate Relationship Humans Have with Sugar

Sugar's allure is undeniable. From the minute we are born, we are physically designed to seek sweetness. Breast milk, the first food for most humans, is naturally sweet, giving critical nutrients and a pleasant flavor. As we grow, sweet foods become a source of pleasure and reward. Birthday cakes, Christmas cookies, and celebratory treats symbolize our milestones and special occasions. These wonderful events are engraved into our memories, cementing the emotional link we have with sweets.

Yet, this love affair with sugar is laden with inconsistencies. As much as we pleasure in its taste, we are increasingly conscious of its potential risks. Public health campaigns and scientific investigations have called attention to the detrimental implications of excessive sugar consumption. We are encouraged to cut back, to read labels more carefully, to be watchful about hidden sugars. This knowledge produces a tension, a push and pull between want and restraint, indulgence and discipline.

The dichotomy lies in our simultaneous need for and hatred of sugar. We blame it as the fundamental cause of many modern health crises, yet we cannot seem to escape its pull. The food business exploits this ambivalence, offering items that appeal to our basic appetites while selling them as healthy or low-sugar solutions. This dichotomy is evident in the way we consume sugar: with both guilt and gratification.

Brief History of Sugar Use and Its Increasing Scrutiny

The history of sugar is a narrative of exploration, exploitation, and economic revolution. Sugarcane, the plant from which most table sugar is derived, was initially domesticated in New Guinea circa 8000 BCE. From then, it went to India, where the technology of turning sugarcane juice into crystalline sugar was created. This "khanda," the Sanskrit word for sugar, is the origin of the word "candy."

Sugar reached the Western world through the conquests of Alexander the Great, who brought it back to Greece from India. However, it was not until the Arab invasion in the 7th century that sugar cultivation and processing extended over the Middle East, North Africa, and eventually into Europe. By the Middle Ages, sugar had become a highly desired luxury item in Europe, frequently referred to as "white gold" due to its rarity and expense.

The demand for sugar increased in the 16th and 17th centuries, coinciding with the colonization of the Americas. European powers created large sugar plantations in the Caribbean and South America, relying on the labor of enslaved Africans. This terrible episode in history shows the human cost of sugar extraction, with millions of lives sacrificed or irreversibly damaged by the brutal circumstances on sugar plantations.

By the 18th century, sugar had become more economical and available, leading to its inclusion in common meals. This period witnessed the introduction of sweetened beverages like tea, coffee, and hot chocolate, which fuelled the demand for sugar even more. The Industrial Revolution brought substantial breakthroughs in sugar refining and distribution, establishing its role as a staple in the Western diet.

The 20th century marked a turning point in the perspective of sugar. Post-World War II, the food industry enjoyed a boom, leading to the widespread manufacture of processed goods. Sugar, with its capacity to enhance flavor and preserve shelf life, became a vital ingredient in a wide array of products. However, the growth in sugar consumption matched a surge in diet-related health disorders, encouraging scientists and health professionals to explore its consequences more closely.

In the 1970s, pioneering research began to link high sugar intake with obesity, diabetes, and heart disease. These findings were first met with resistance, particularly from the sugar industry, which undertook vigorous campaigns to discredit the research and shift the attention to dietary fats as the key culprit in health problems. Despite these attempts, the volume of evidence against sugar continues to expand.

The 21st century has seen an intensification of attention on sugar. Public health agencies, such as the World Health Organization and the Centers for Disease Control and Prevention, have released guidelines advocating lower sugar intake. Governments have introduced measures like sugar tariffs and stricter labeling regulations to curb consumption. These efforts indicate an increasing realization of the need to address the health hazards linked with excessive sugar consumption.

The cultural shift in attitudes about sugar is also visible in consumer behavior. More individuals are searching out "sugar-free" or "reduced sugar" items, and there is a heightened awareness of the presence of hidden sugars in processed meals. This has led to an increase in demand for natural sweeteners and alternatives, such as stevia, monk fruit, and erythritol.

However, the struggle against sugar is far from done. The food business continues to innovate, creating new formulations that cater to both the demand for sweetness and the desire for healthier solutions. This continuing change creates both obstacles and possibilities for customers striving to make educated choices.

The scrutiny of sugar extends beyond health issues to its larger socioeconomic and environmental implications. The cultivation of sugarcane and sugar beets consumes enormous resources, often leading to deforestation, soil depletion, and water shortages. Additionally, the working conditions on current sugar plantations, while improved from the days of slavery, nonetheless present ethical problems concerning labor rights and fair remuneration.

Understanding the complicated history and contemporary dynamics of sugar consumption is vital for navigating the modern dietary landscape. By exploring the connection between biology, culture, and industry, we can obtain a deeper comprehension of why sugar occupies such a powerful role in our lives. This information helps us to make decisions that balance our love of sweetness with our health and well-being.

As we move forward, it is vital to continue evaluating the role of sugar in our diets and culture. This entails not only personal decisions about what we eat but also societal activities to address the broader implications of sugar production and consumption. The journey towards a healthier relationship with sugar is continual, needing vigilance, education, and a willingness to challenge previous preconceptions.

The love-hate relationship with sugar is a reflection of our greater difficulties with diet and health. It illustrates the struggle between indulgence and control, pleasure and caution. By investigating this paradox, we can begin to grasp the various motivations and forces that determine our eating choices. This understanding is the first step in achieving a more balanced and educated approach to sugar consumption.

Purpose: Explanation of Why This Book is Necessary

In a world where dietary standards and health advice appear to change almost daily, there is an urgent need for clear, evidence-based information concerning sugar. The landscape of modern nutrition is filled with contradicting signals, frequently leaving consumers confused and overwhelmed. This uncertainty is particularly obvious when it comes to sugar, a ubiquitous component that has been the focal focus of considerable controversy. The necessity of this book rests in its objective to cut through the noise, presenting readers with a balanced understanding of sugar's function in our diets and its impact on our health.

The demonization of sugar has led to widespread beliefs that can influence our dietary patterns and health choices. Many people have embraced extreme measures, such as completely removing sugar from their diets, without fully comprehending the scientific basis for their choices or the potential implications. Others continue to consume sugar-laden foods without awareness of the risks, lured into a false feeling of security by misleading marketing. This book is vital to bridge this knowledge gap, presenting a balanced perspective that helps readers to make informed judgments.

Sugar is more than just a food component; it is firmly interwoven in our cultural traditions, economic institutions, and personal lives. The complications of sugar consumption extend beyond human health to broader societal and environmental ramifications. Addressing these concerns requires a holistic approach that examines the historical backdrop, scientific data, and practical measures for managing sugar intake. This book strives to provide that complete view, helping readers to negotiate the complexity of sugar consumption with confidence and clarity.

The increasing prevalence of diet-related disorders such as obesity, diabetes, and heart disease underline the necessity of understanding the components that contribute to these conditions. While sugar is not the primary problem, it is a substantial contributor that merits serious consideration. By examining the myths and facts of sugar consumption, this book strives to inform public health debate and promote healthy eating behaviors. It serves as a vital resource for individuals, families, healthcare professionals, and policymakers seeking to tackle the health concerns of our time.

Additionally, this book covers the ethical and environmental implications of sugar production. The history of sugar is defined by exploitation and inequality, with lasting repercussions that continue to echo today. Understanding these components is vital for making conscientious decisions that accord with both personal health goals and broader social and environmental concerns. This book illustrates these interconnected challenges, encouraging a better knowledge of the true cost of sugar.

The necessity of this book resides in its commitment to giving clear, balanced, and actionable information regarding sugar. It strives to dispel myths, clarify misconceptions, and educate readers toward better, more informed choices. By addressing the multidimensional nature of sugar consumption, this book offers a complete resource that is both contemporary and vital in the ongoing quest for better health and well-being.

Overview: Brief Introduction to What Will Be Covered in the Book

This book is organized to offer a detailed and insightful investigation of sugar from numerous aspects, giving readers a well-rounded grasp of this complicated issue. It begins by establishing the foundations with a core understanding of sugar, including its origins, kinds, and the procedures involved in its manufacture. This opening section lays the framework for a deeper dive into the science and history of sugar, building a solid base of information that will be built upon throughout the book.

Following the introductory material, the book addresses the biochemical and physiological implications of sugar ingestion. Readers will learn about how sugar is processed in the body, its function in energy production, and the immediate and long-term implications of sugar intake on health. This part gives a deep look at the scientific principles that support our understanding of sugar, demystifying complex processes in a way that is approachable and entertaining.

The book then shifts to a study of the myths around sugar. These chapters critically explore widespread misconceptions about sugar and its alleged effects, such as its link to weight gain, diabetes, hyperactivity, and addiction. Each myth is analyzed using data from scientific studies, presenting a balanced perspective that challenges simple tales. This section attempts to empower readers with the information to separate fact from fiction, creating a more informed approach to sugar consumption.

Moving from myth-busting to practical assistance, the book gives solutions for managing sugar intake in daily life. Readers will learn practical techniques for recognizing hidden sugars in processed goods, making healthier dietary choices, and consuming sugar in a balanced way. This section also contains recommendations for natural sweeteners and alternatives, helping readers explore the multitude of options available. Recipes and culinary ideas provide real tools for decreasing sugar without compromising flavor, making it easier to adopt healthy habits.

The book also addresses the broader societal and environmental repercussions of sugar production and use. It analyzes the history of the sugar trade, the impact of sugar plantations, and the ongoing concerns connected to labor rights and environmental sustainability. This section connects personal food decisions to wider global challenges, prompting readers to evaluate the ethical elements of their consumption.

Throughout the book, real-life anecdotes and case studies exemplify the issues presented, bringing a human flavor to the scientific and historical study. These anecdotes emphasize the different ways in which sugar influences individual lives, presenting relatable instances that appeal to readers.

This book covers a wide range of themes relating to sugar, from its biochemical qualities and health impacts to its cultural significance and ethical considerations. Each component is designed to build on the preceding one, producing a cohesive and complete resource that gives readers the knowledge and tools to make informed decisions about sugar consumption.

Why This Matters: Highlight the Impact of Sugar Myths on Health and Well-Being

The persistent beliefs around sugar have far-reaching effects on our health and well-being. Misconceptions about sugar can lead to poor food choices, erroneous health practices, and a skewed view of nutrition. Addressing these fallacies is not only an academic exercise; it is a critical step toward improving public health and individual quality of life.

One of the most pernicious fallacies is the belief that sugar is the primary cause of obesity. While sugar contributes to weight gain when ingested in excess, it is simply one element of a much broader puzzle. The oversimplification of sugar as the single villain distracts from other crucial aspects such as total calorie intake, physical exercise, and overall dietary patterns. This narrow emphasis might lead to inefficient or severe dietary changes that fail to address the core causes of obesity.

The belief that sugars directly causes diabetes is another example of how myths can affect our understanding of health. While high sugar intake is connected with an increased risk of acquiring type 2 diabetes, the relationship is not as straightforward as typically described. Factors such as genetics, lifestyle, and overall diet play a crucial influence in the development of diabetes. Simplifying the story to "sugar equals diabetes" might lead to undue fear and restricted eating patterns that may not be good in the long term.

Hyperactivity in children is another area where sugar misconceptions have taken root. Many parents believe that sugar consumption contributes to hyperactive behavior, despite scientific evidence indicating no consistent link between the two. This idea can impact parenting techniques and eating choices, frequently leading to unwarranted limitations that do not address the true reasons for behavioral difficulties.

Understanding the true effects of sugar will help parents make more informed decisions about their children's meals and overall health.

The notion of sugar addiction is a particularly ubiquitous myth that impacts how individuals interpret their relationship with food. While desires for sweet foods are typical, associating these cravings with addiction can produce a sense of helplessness and guilt. This perspective can hamper efforts to establish healthier eating habits by presenting the issue as a lack of willpower rather than a matter of balanced nutrition. Recognizing the distinction between cravings and addiction is vital for creating effective techniques to limit sugar intake.

Beyond individual health, sugar myths also affect public health policies and activities. Misguided ideas about sugar can influence the course of health campaigns, leading to policies that may not adequately address the intricacies of diet-related disorders. For example, focusing simply on reducing sugar intake without considering other dietary and lifestyle factors can result in incomplete or inefficient health interventions. A more sophisticated understanding of sugar's function in health is important for designing comprehensive public health interventions.

The societal influence of sugar myths extends to the food industry and consumer behavior. Misleading marketing strategies capitalize on these fallacies, promoting "sugar-free" or "low-sugar" products that may not be healthier overall. Consumers who are misled by these assertions may make choices that do not fit with their health goals. Educating consumers about the realities of sugar can help them navigate the marketplace more successfully and choose choices that promote their well-being.

The environmental and ethical implications of sugar production are also influenced by misconceptions. Romanticized conceptions of sugar's harmlessness can hide the harsh reality of its manufacturing, including labor exploitation and environmental devastation. Raising knowledge about these concerns is vital for encouraging more ethical and sustainable consumption patterns. Consumers who are aware of the larger implications of sugar should lobby for reforms in the industry and support more responsible manufacturing techniques.

The cumulative result of sugar myths is a distorted picture of diet and health that inhibits progress toward better lives. By exposing these beliefs and presenting accurate information, this book strives to address these misconceptions and promote a more balanced and informed attitude toward sugar consumption. This shift in perspective is critical for improving individual health outcomes, influencing public health policy, and building a more sustainable and ethical food system.

Understanding the true impact of sugar and differentiating fact from myth is crucial for empowering individuals to take control of their health. By refuting myths and giving evidence-based insights, this book gives readers the knowledge they need to make informed nutritional decisions. This informed approach is not only excellent for personal health but also contributes to a broader cultural movement toward more ethical and sustainable purchasing patterns. The importance of tackling sugar myths cannot be emphasized, since it is a critical step in promoting general well-being and ensuring a healthy future for all.

Chapter 1

What is table sugar

Table sugar, commonly known as sucrose, is a disaccharide comprised of glucose and fructose. Sucrose is a naturally occurring carbohydrate present in many plants, mainly in sugarcane and sugar beets. It is the most recognizable kind of sugar and is widely used in households and food production for its sweetness and capacity to enhance flavor and texture in many meals and beverages.

Sugarcane and sugar beets are the principal sources of table sugar. Sugarcane is a tropical grass that grows in warm areas, while sugar beets are a root crop that flourishes in cooler, temperate settings. Both plants contain sucrose in their tissues, which may be extracted and refined to make the white, crystalline sugar that is prevalent in kitchens around the world.

The sweetness of table sugar makes it a versatile ingredient in culinary applications. It not only offers sweetness but also plays a part in browning events during baking, protects foods by limiting microbial development, and helps the texture and mouthfeel of items like sweets and ice cream. Because of its multipurpose features, table sugar is a mainstay in both home cooking and industrial food manufacturing.

What is the Manufacturing Process of Table Sugar?

The manufacturing of table sugar comprises multiple phases, from harvesting the raw materials to refining the end product. The process begins with the planting and harvesting of sugarcane or sugar beets.

1. Harvesting:

Sugarcane is often harvested by cutting the stalks close to the ground, either manually with machetes or mechanically using harvesters. The collected stalks are taken to mills for processing. Sugar beets are pulled from the ground using specialized machinery, cleaned, and then transported to processing plants.

2. Extraction:

Once at the mill, sugarcane stalks are washed and diced into small pieces to assist juice extraction. The chopped cane is run through a series of crushing mills or diffusers to extract the juice. The residual fibrous material, termed bagasse, is commonly utilized as a biofuel or in paper manufacture. In the instance of sugar beets, the beets are cut into thin strips called cassettes. These strips are subsequently processed in a diffuser, where hot water removes the sugar from the beet slices.

3. Clarification:

The extracted juice from both sugarcane and sugar beets contains contaminants such as plant fibers, dirt, and other organic elements. To remove these contaminants, the juice undergoes a clarifying procedure. Lime (calcium hydroxide) is added to the juice, which interacts with the contaminants to generate insoluble compounds.

These chemicals are subsequently removed by filtration or sedimentation, leaving a clear juice.

4. Concentration:

The clarified juice is concentrated by boiling it in evaporators to get rid of surplus water. This results in a thick syrup termed "thick juice" in beet processing and "concentrated juice" in cane processing. This syrup has a high sugar concentration but still contains certain contaminants.

5. Crystallization:

The concentrated juice is further evaporated in vacuum pans to supersaturate the solution and produce crystallization. Sugar crystals begin to form as the fluid cools. This blend of sugar crystals and syrup is called massecuite. The massecuite is next spun in centrifugal machines to separate the sugar crystals from the leftover syrup, known as molasses. The sugar crystals are cleaned with water or steam to eliminate any leftover contaminants.

6. Refining:

The raw sugar crystals produced in the initial crystallization process are not yet pure white table sugar. They undergo further refining to reach the necessary purity and whiteness. The raw sugar is dissolved in hot water to make a syrup, which is then treated with phosphoric acid and calcium hydroxide to precipitate impurities. The syrup is filtered via activated carbon or bone char to remove colorants and residual impurities. The purified syrup is then evaporated and crystallized once more to yield refined sugar crystals.

7. Drying and Packaging:

The final stage entails drying the refined sugar crystals to minimize clumping and produce a free-flowing product. The dried sugar is next screened to separate any oversized or undersized crystals. The completed sugar is packaged into various forms, such as granulated sugar, powdered sugar, and sugar cubes, ready for distribution and consumption.

What is the Nutritional Value of Table Sugar?

Table sugar, or sucrose, is a source of energy but provides no substantial nutritional benefits beyond its caloric value. It has 4 calories per gram, making it a rich source of energy. However, it lacks critical elements such as vitamins, minerals, protein, and fiber. As a result, it is commonly referred to as "empty calories."

When ingested, sucrose is broken down into its constituent monosaccharides, glucose, and fructose, which are subsequently absorbed into the bloodstream. Glucose is a key energy source for the body's cells, while fructose is processed predominantly in the liver.

While table sugar can give a rapid source of energy, excessive use is related to different health concerns. High intake of added sugars has been associated with obesity, type 2 diabetes, heart disease, and dental cavities. The American Heart Association recommends reducing added sugar intake to no more than 6 teaspoons (25 grams) per day for women and 9 teaspoons (38 grams) per day for men to lower the risk of certain health concerns.

Despite its lack of nutrients, sugar can be a part in a balanced diet when consumed in moderation. It is vital to differentiate between naturally occurring sugars found in fruits, vegetables, and dairy products, which come with critical nutrients and added sugars, which give additional calories without nutritional advantages.

Which Chemicals Being Used in the Making of Table Sugar?

The manufacturing of table sugar requires numerous chemicals and substances that aid in the extraction, purification, and refinement processes. These compounds are used to ensure the efficiency and quality of sugar manufacturing, resulting in a pure and safe product for consumption.

1. Lime (Calcium Hydroxide):

Lime is used throughout the clarifying process to eliminate contaminants from the sugar juice. When added to the juice, lime reacts with organic and inorganic contaminants, generating insoluble molecules that may be filtered away. This stage aids in producing a clear juice that is required for further processing.

2. Carbon Dioxide:

In some sugar refining processes, carbon dioxide is utilized in combination with lime in a stage called carbonation. Carbon dioxide combines with the calcium hydroxide to generate calcium carbonate, which helps to trap and remove contaminants. This technique significantly clarifies the juice before crystallization.

3. Phosphoric Acid:

Phosphoric acid is sometimes used in the purifying process of sugar refining. It helps to precipitate contaminants and colorants, making it easier to filter them out. The use of phosphoric acid contributes to getting the necessary purity and color of the final sugar product.

4. Activated Carbon or Bone Char:

Activated carbon and bone char are employed as filtration media to remove colorants and residual contaminants from the sugar syrup. These chemicals have significant adsorption capabilities, effectively trapping undesirable molecules and contributing to the decolorization of the sugar. Bone char, derived from animal bones, is a traditional approach, whereas activated carbon, made from diverse carbon-rich sources, is a modern option.

5. Sulfur Dioxide:

Sulfur dioxide is employed in various sugar manufacturing processes as a bleaching agent. It helps to brighten the color of the sugar syrup, resulting in a whiter end product. The usage of sulfur dioxide must be carefully managed to ensure that any residues in the finished product remain within safe limits.

6. Polyacrylamide:

Polyacrylamide is a flocculant used in the clarifying process to assist remove suspended particulates from the juice. It stimulates the agglomeration of tiny particles, making them easier to filter out. This stage boosts the clarity of the juice, helping the overall efficiency of the sugar extraction process.

7. Lime Kiln Dust:

In some sugar production facilities, lime kiln dust, a byproduct of lime manufacture, is utilized as an alternative to lime. It contains calcium oxide, which has a similar function in the clarifying process, helping to eliminate contaminants from the sugar juice.

8. Antifoaming Agents:

During the boiling and evaporation stages, foam might form, which can hamper the effectiveness of the operation. Antifoaming chemicals, such as polydimethylsiloxane or vegetable oils, are used to prevent the production of foam, assuring smooth and efficient operation.

9. Ion Exchange Resins:

Ion exchange resins are employed in several sugar refining procedures to remove specific ions and contaminants from the sugar syrup. These resins aid the filtration of the syrup by exchanging unwanted ions with innocuous ones, improving the overall quality of the finished product.

The usage of these chemicals and compounds in the manufacturing of table sugar is rigorously regulated to assure the safety and quality of the finished product. The methods are meant to remove impurities and pollutants, resulting in pure, white sugar that passes food safety standards. It is crucial to note that while these chemicals are employed during production, the end product contains only minimal, if any, residues of these substances, making it safe for eating.

Understanding the manufacturing process and the chemicals involved helps to demystify the creation of table sugar. It also illustrates the precision and care necessary to manufacture a product that is both safe and consistent in quality.

Is There Any Alternative to Table Sugar?

In recent years, the demand for alternatives to table sugar has increased, driven by growing health concerns and the desire for more natural and lower-calorie solutions. Several alternatives to table sugar have been created, each with its distinct qualities, benefits, and potential concerns.

1. Natural Sweeteners:

Natural sweeteners are sourced from plants and provide a sweet taste without the calories or blood sugar rises associated with table sugar.

Honey: Honey is a natural sweetener created by bees from the nectar of flowers. It contains modest levels of vitamins, minerals, and antioxidants, making it a better option than table sugar. Honey is sugary than sugar, thus less is needed to get the same amount of sweetness. However, it is high in fructose and can influence blood sugar levels, therefore it should be used in moderation.

Maple Syrup: Maple syrup is created from the sap of sugar maple trees. It contains antioxidants and minerals like calcium, potassium, and zinc. Maple syrup has a lower glycemic index than table sugar, suggesting it has a less dramatic influence on blood sugar levels. However, it is still heavy in sugar and should be taken sparingly.

Agave Nectar: Agave nectar is from agave plant. It has a low glycemic index, which means it promotes a slower rise in blood sugar levels. However, agave nectar is high in fructose, which can be toxic in large amounts and may contribute to insulin resistance and fatty liver disease if consumed excessively.

Stevia: Stevia is a natural sweetener extracted from the leaves of the Stevia rebaudiana plant. It is sugary than sugar and has zero calories. Stevia does not elevate blood sugar levels, making it a popular choice for persons with diabetes and those trying to lower their calorie intake. Some people may notice that it has a little harsh aftertaste.

2. Sugar Alcohols:

Sugar alcohols are a form of carbohydrate that exists naturally in various fruits and vegetables but can also be produced. They are widely employed as sweeteners in sugar-free and reduced-calorie products.

Xylitol: Xylitol is a sugar alcohol that is as sweet as sugar but has fewer calories. It does not produce a sudden increase in blood sugar levels and is safe for those with diabetes. Xylitol also has dental benefits, as it can help reduce tooth decay. However, drinking big amounts might induce digestive difficulties like bloating and diarrhea.

Erythritol: Erythritol is a sugar alcohol that has around 70% of the sweetness of sugar and nearly no calories. It does not raise blood sugar or insulin levels and is generally well-tolerated. Erythritol is less prone to produce digestive troubles compared to other sugar alcohols, but excessive use can still lead to discomfort.

Sorbitol: Sorbitol is a sugar alcohol that is about 60% as sweet as sugar and has fewer calories. It is widely used in sugar-free candies and chewing gum. Sorbitol has a low glycemic index but can induce digestive difficulties, such as gas and diarrhea when ingested in high quantities.

3. Artificial Sweeteners:

Artificial sweeteners are synthetic chemicals that deliver sweetness without the calories of sugar. They are often used in diet drinks, sugar-free goods, and as table sweeteners.

Aspartame: Aspartame is a low-calorie sweetener that is around 200 times sweeter than sugar. It is widely found in diet sodas, sugar-free gum, and other low-calorie goods. Aspartame is safe for most individuals, however, those with phenylketonuria (PKU) should avoid it, as they cannot metabolize phenylalanine, a component of aspartame.

Sucralose: Sucralose is an artificial sweetener that is round 600 times sweeter than sugar and has no calories. It is heat-stable, making it perfect for baking and cooking. Sucralose is usually regarded as safe;

however, some research suggests it may affect gut microbes and impair glucose metabolism.

Saccharin: Saccharin is an artificial sweetener that is 300-400 times sweeter than sugar and has no calories. It has been used for almost a century and is used in numerous sugar-free goods. Saccharin was originally related to cancer in animal experiments, but further study has found it to be safe for human intake.

4. Novel Sweeteners:

Novel sweeteners are novel and developing solutions that combine the benefits of natural and artificial sweeteners.

Monk Fruit Extract: Monk fruit extract is a natural sweetener obtained from the monk fruit. It is around 150-200 times sweeter than sugar and contains no calories. Monk fruit extract does not raise blood sugar levels and is generally well-tolerated, with no documented negative effects.

Allulose: Allulose is a rare sugar found naturally in small quantities in fruits like figs and raisins. It has roughly 70% of the sweetness of sugar and on a fraction of the calories. Allulose does not significantly alter blood sugar levels and is well-tolerated by most people, however, excessive use can cause stomach discomfort.

How Much Sugar is Safe to Consume?

Determining the safe amount of sugar to ingest is vital for maintaining good health and preventing diet-related disorders. The recommendations for sugar intake vary based on the source, but numerous principles can assist in establishing a foundation for appropriate consumption.

The American Heart Association (AHA) recommends that women restrict their intake of added sugars to no more than 6 teaspoons (25 grams) per day and men to no more than 9 teaspoons (38 grams) per day. These limitations are aimed at lowering the risk of cardiovascular disease, obesity, and other health concerns linked with high sugar consumption.

The World Health Organization (WHO) says that added sugars should make up less than 10% of total daily calorie consumption, with a further reduction to below

5% having additional health benefits. For an average adult with a 2,000-calorie diet, this amounts to no more than 50 grams of added sugar per day, with an optimal limit of 25 grams.

These guidelines focus on added sugars, which are sugars and syrups added to foods and beverages during manufacturing or preparation. This includes sugars added to products like sodas, sweets, pastries, and other processed foods. Naturally occurring sugars found in fruits, vegetables, and dairy products are not included in these restrictions, as they come with necessary nutrients and fiber.

Exceeding these advised levels can have major health repercussions. High sugar intake is connected with an increased risk of obesity, type 2 diabetes, heart disease, and dental cavities. Excessive sugar consumption can lead to weight gain by contributing to a higher overall calorie intake without giving satisfaction. This can result in an imbalance between energy intake and expenditure, leading to fat buildup and obesity.

In addition to weight gain, increased sugar intake might damage metabolic health. Consuming significant amounts of sugar, particularly in the form of sugary beverages, can lead to insulin resistance, a condition where the body's cells become less receptive to insulin. This can eventually lead to type 2 diabetes, a chronic condition characterized by high blood sugar levels and associated with many complications such as nerve damage, renal disease, and cardiovascular difficulties.

High sugar consumption is also connected to an increased risk of heart disease. Diets heavy in added sugars can elevate blood pressure, cause inflammation, and contribute to unhealthy cholesterol levels, all of which are risk factors for cardiovascular disease. Reducing sugar intake can assist improve heart health and minimize the risk of heart attacks and strokes.

Dental health is another area influenced by sugar consumption. Sugars produce a food source for bacteria in the mouth, which produce acids that can erode tooth enamel and lead to cavities. Reducing sugar intake and keeping appropriate oral hygiene practices are vital for preventing dental decay and preserving general oral health.

Is There Any Health Benefits of Taking Table Sugar?

While table sugar is typically criticized for its negative health consequences, it is vital to realize that it can also give certain benefits when ingested in moderation. Understanding these benefits might help place sugar in a more balanced context within a healthy diet.

1. Quick Source of Energy:

Table sugar, or sucrose, is a carbohydrate that provides a quick source of energy. When ingested, it is broken down into glucose and fructose, which are taken into the bloodstream. Glucose is the main energy source for the body's cells, mostly for the brain and muscles. This makes sugar excellent for providing a rapid energy boost, especially during moments of high physical activity or mental exertion.

2. Enhances Flavor and Palatability:

Sugar is frequently used in cooking and baking to increase the flavor and palatability of foods. It not only offers sweetness but also balances the flavors of other ingredients, lowering bitterness and enriching the overall taste experience. This can encourage the eating of nutrient-dense meals that might otherwise be less enticing.

3. Preservation of Food:

Sugar has been used as a preservative for ages. It inhibits the growth of bacteria by reducing the water activity in foods, which helps prevent spoiling and lengthen shelf life. This feature is particularly helpful in the preservation of jams, jellies, and other canned goods, allowing for the long-term storage of seasonal produce.

4. Improvement of Texture and Structure:

In baking and confection, sugar contributes to the texture and structure of products. It helps generate the light, fluffy texture of cakes and the chewiness of cookies. Sugar also plays a part in the browning events during baking, such as the Maillard reaction and caramelization, which enhance the color and flavor of baked goods.

5. Social and Cultural Importance:

Sugar has great social and cultural relevance. It is commonly utilized in festive foods and rituals, playing a prominent role in holidays, festivals, and family gatherings. The pleasure of sweet foods can build social relationships and contribute to favorable emotional experiences.

While these benefits show the significance of sugar in numerous elements of cuisine and culture, it is vital to consume it in moderation to prevent the potential negative health effects associated with excessive intake.

What are the Side Effects of Consuming Table Sugar?

Despite its benefits, excessive use of table sugar can lead to a range of unfavorable health effects. Understanding these hazards is vital for making informed dietary choices and sustaining overall health.

1. Weight Gain and Obesity:

One of the most well-documented negative effects of heavy sugar intake is weight gain. Sugary foods and beverages are generally high in calories but low in satiety, leading to increased overall calorie consumption. Excess calories are deposited as fat, resulting in weight gain and obesity. Obesity, in turn, is a substantial risk factor for various health issues, including heart disease, type 2 diabetes, and some malignancies.

2. Insulin Resistance and Type 2 Diabetes:

Regular ingestion of significant amounts of sugar, particularly in the form of sugary drinks, can lead to insulin resistance. Insulin resistance occurs when the body's cells become less receptive to insulin, leading the pancreas to produce more insulin to maintain normal blood sugar levels. Over time, this might tire the pancreas and lead to type 2 diabetes. Type 2 diabetes is a chronic disorder characterized by high blood sugar levels and associated with consequences such as neuropathy, renal disease, and cardiovascular difficulties.

3.Heart disease:

High sugar intake is connected to an increased risk of heart disease. Diets strong in added sugars can contribute to increased blood pressure, higher triglycerides, and low levels of HDL (good) cholesterol, all of which are risk factors for cardiovascular disease. Additionally, high sugar consumption can contribute to chronic inflammation, further raising the risk of heart disease.

4. Dental Cavities:

Sugars provide a food source for bacteria in the mouth, that produce acids that can erode tooth enamel and lead to cavities. Frequent consumption of sugary foods and drinks raises the risk of dental decay, particularly if basic oral hygiene is not maintained. Reducing sugar intake and maintaining proper oral hygiene can help avoid cavities and maintain dental health.

5. Non-Alcoholic Fatty Liver Disease (NAFLD):

High consumption of fructose, a component of table sugar, has connected with non-alcoholic fatty liver disease (NAFLD). Fructose is processed predominantly in the liver, where it can be turned into fat. Excessive fructose intake can lead to fat deposition in the liver, contributing to NAFLD. This disorder can progress to more serious liver diseases, such as non-alcoholic steatohepatitis (NASH), cirrhosis, and liver cancer.

6. Increased Risk of Certain Cancers:

Some studies suggest that high sugar intake may be associated with an increased risk of some malignancies, such as breast, colon, and pancreatic cancer. While the underlying mechanisms are not entirely understood, it is believed that excessive sugar consumption might induce inflammation, insulin resistance, and obesity, all of which are risk factors for cancer development.

7. Mental Health and Cognitive Function:

Emerging evidence reveals that increased sugar intake may have harmful impacts on mental health and cognitive performance. Diets high in added sugars have been connected with an increased risk of depression, anxiety, and cognitive deterioration. While further research is needed to grasp these associations thoroughly, it is hypothesized that the inflammatory effects of sugar and its impact on blood sugar regulation may play a role.

8. Skin Aging:

Excessive sugar consumption can hasten skin aging through a process called glycation. Glycation occurs when sugar molecules connect to proteins in the skin, generating advanced glycation end-products (AGEs). AGEs can damage collagen and elastin, proteins that maintain skin's firmness and elasticity, resulting in wrinkles and drooping skin. Reducing sugar intake can help retain skin health and prevent the effects of aging.

9. Addiction and Cravings:

Sugar can have addictive characteristics, leading to cravings and overconsumption. The ingestion of sugar causes the production of dopamine, a neurotransmitter associated with pleasure and reward, in the brain. This can generate a loop of need and consumption, comparable to the effects of addictive substances.

Managing sugar intake might help interrupt this pattern and promote healthier eating habits.

Recognizing the potential adverse effects of excessive sugar consumption underscores the significance of moderation and balanced dietary choices. By understanding the risks, individuals may make informed decisions about their sugar intake and take steps to protect their health and well-being.

Definition and Types of Sugar (Sucrose, Fructose, Glucose) vs. Added Sugars

Natural Sugars:

Sucrose: Sucrose is widely known as table sugar and is a disaccharide, meaning it is made of two monosaccharides: glucose and fructose. Sucrose is certainly found in many plants, mainly in sugar cane and sugar beets, from which it is routinely harvested and refined for use as table sugar. It is also prevalent in fruits and vegetables.

Fructose: Fructose, also referred to as fruit sugar, is a monosaccharide found naturally in fruits, honey, and some root vegetables. It is the sweetest of all-natural sugars. Fructose is commonly utilized in the food business, often in the form of high-fructose corn syrup (HFCS), which is a combination of fructose and glucose generated from maize starch.

Glucose: Glucose is a monosaccharide and a main source of energy for the body's cells. It is found in fruits, vegetables, and honey. Glucose is less sweet than fructose and is also a component of different carbohydrates, including starches and other sugars. When carbs are consumed, they are broken down into glucose during digestion.

Added Sugars:

Added sugars are sugars and syrups that are added to foods and beverages throughout processing or preparation. These are not naturally occurring sugars found in entire foods. Common sources of added sugars include sodas, sweets, baked goods, and sweetened dairy products.

Added sugars might be in the form of sucrose, high-fructose corn syrup, or alternative sweeteners like honey and agave syrup. The fundamental worry with added sugars is their contribution to increased calorie intake without delivering important nutrients, resulting in different health conditions such as obesity, diabetes, and heart disease.

Chemical Structure and Properties

Sucrose: The chemical formula for sucrose is $C_{12}H_{22}O_{11}$. It is a disaccharide comprised of one molecule of glucose and one molecule of fructose connected by a glycosidic bond. Sucrose is extremely soluble in water and has a pleasant taste. Its crystalline form makes it perfect for different culinary uses, including baking and confectionery.

Fructose: Fructose has the chemical formula $C_6H_{12}O_6$. It is a monosaccharide having a five-membered ring structure, different from the six-membered ring structure of glucose. Fructose is extremely soluble in water and is the sweetest of all-natural sugars, making it a common sweetener in processed foods and beverages.

Glucose: Glucose also has the molecular formula $C_6H_{12}O_6$. It is a monosaccharide having a six-membered ring structure. Glucose is less sweet than fructose and is a key energy source for the body. It is extremely soluble in water and plays a critical function in different metabolic processes.

Added Sugars: Added sugars can vary in chemical structure depending on the type of sugar used. Common added sugars include sucrose, high-fructose corn syrup (which contains various ratios of glucose and fructose), and glucose syrups. These sugars are frequently added to enhance the flavor, texture, and shelf life of processed foods and beverages.

How Sugar is Metabolized

Sugar metabolism involves a set of metabolic reactions that turn sugars into energy for the body's cells. This process begins with the digestion of carbohydrates in the food and continues through several metabolic pathways in the body.

1. Digestion: The digestion of sugars starts in the mouth when salivary amylase begins breaking down complex carbohydrates into simpler sugars. This process continues in the small intestine, where enzymes including sucrase, lactase, and maltase further break down disaccharides and polysaccharides into monosaccharides (glucose, fructose, and galactose).

2. Absorption: Once broken down into monosaccharides, these sugars are absorbed via the intestinal lining and reach the bloodstream. Glucose and galactose are taken via active transport pathways using sodium-glucose transport proteins, while fructose is absorbed through facilitated diffusion using specialized fructose transporters.

3. Utilization: After absorption, monosaccharides are delivered to the liver via the portal vein. In the liver, fructose, and galactose are transformed into glucose or other metabolites by different enzyme processes.

Glucose can be used instantly for energy, stored as glycogen in the liver and muscles, or transformed into fat for long-term energy storage.

Digestion, Absorption, and Utilization of Sugar

1. Digestion:

Mouth: The digestion of carbohydrates begins in the mouth with the enzyme salivary amylase, which breaks down starches into smaller polysaccharides and maltose. However, this process is rather brief, as food immediately goes to the stomach where the acidic environment inactivates amylase.

Stomach: In the stomach, the acidic environment halts carbohydrate digestion, as the enzymes involved in breaking down sugars are not active in acidic circumstances. However, mechanical digestion continues as the stomach churns food into a semi-liquid form known as chyme.

Small Intestine: The majority of carbohydrate digestion happens in the small intestine. Pancreatic amylase, released from the pancreas, continues to break down polysaccharides into disaccharides. Specific enzymes found on the surface of the intestinal lining (brush boundary enzymes) further break down disaccharides into monosaccharides. Sucrase breaks down sucrose in glucose and fructose, lactase breaks down lactose into glucose and galactose, and maltase breaks down maltose into two glucose molecules.

2. Absorption:

The absorption of monosaccharides happens largely in the small intestine.

Glucose and Galactose: These sugars are absorbed by active transport pathways involving sodium-glucose co-transporters (SGLT1). This process takes energy, as it entails the transport of glucose and galactose against their concentration gradients. Once inside the intestinal cells, glucose and galactose moved into the bloodstream via facilitated diffusion via glucose transporters (GLUT2).

Fructose: Fructose is absorbed through facilitated diffusion using a particular fructose transporter (GLUT5). This process does not require energy, as fructose goes down its concentration gradient. Once absorbed, fructose is taken into the circulation and delivered to the liver for processing.

3. Utilization:

Liver Metabolism: Once absorbed, monosaccharides are delivered to the liver via the portal vein. In the liver, fructose, and galactose are transformed into glucose or other metabolites. Fructose is a very large processed in the liver, where it can be turned into glucose, glycogen, or fat. This process involves numerous enzymatic stages, including phosphorylation by fructokinase and subsequent processing by aldolase B.

Glucose Utilization: Glucose, the primary energy source for the body's cells, is utilized in numerous ways:

Immediate Energy Use: Cells throughout the body take up glucose from the bloodstream and use it for immediate energy production through glycolysis. During glycolysis, glucose is broken down into pyruvate, producing ATP, the main energy currency of the cell.

Glycogen Storage: Much of glucose is stored as glycogen in the liver and muscles. Glycogen can be swiftly mobilized and turned back into glucose when energy is needed, such as during physical exercise or between meals.

Fat Storage: When glycogen stores are full, extra glucose is turned into fat through a process called lipogenesis. This occurs in the liver and adipose tissue, where glucose is transformed into fatty acids and triglycerides for long-term energy storage.

Regulation of Blood Sugar Levels: The body tightly regulates blood glucose levels to guarantee a consistent source of energy. This modulation is done by the actions of insulin and glucagon, chemicals produced by the pancreas. Insulin stimulates the uptake of glucose into cells and promotes glycogen storage, reducing blood sugar levels. Glucagon, on the other hand, increases the breakdown of glycogen and the release of glucose into the bloodstream, boosting blood sugar levels during periods of fasting or low glucose availability.

Metabolic Pathways:

Glycolysis: Glycolysis is the metabolic mechanism that transforms glucose into pyruvate, creating ATP and NADH in the process. This route happens in the cytoplasm of cells and does not require oxygen. Glycolysis is the initial stage in both aerobic and anaerobic respiration, supplying energy for cellular processes.

Glycogenolysis: Glycogenolysis is the process of breaking down glycogen into glucose-1-phosphate, which is then transformed into glucose-6-phosphate and enters the glycolysis pathway. This mechanism occurs in the liver and muscles during periods of fasting or high physical exercise, providing a rapid source of glucose for energy.

Gluconeogenesis: Gluconeogenesis is the metabolic mechanism that creates glucose from non-carbohydrate sources, as amino acids, lactate, and glycerol. This process happens predominantly in the liver and helps sustain blood glucose levels after prolonged fasting or severe physical activity.

Pentose Phosphate Pathway: The pentose phosphate pathway is a metabolic pathway parallel to glycolysis that creates NADPH and ribose-5-phosphate, necessary for biosynthetic reactions and the creation of nucleotides. This pathway is critical for maintaining cellular redox equilibrium and generating precursors for DNA and RNA production.

Understanding the metabolism of sugar, including its digestion, absorption, and utilization, provides insight into how the body processes and uses this crucial nutrient. This knowledge can inform dietary choices and highlight the significance of balancing sugar intake with overall nutritional demands and health goals.

Role of Insulin and Glucose Regulation

Insulin is a hormone made by pancreas that plays a critical role in regulating blood glucose levels and enabling the uptake of glucose into cells for energy production. Proper glucose management is vital for maintaining metabolic balance and general health.

Insulin Production and Release:

When you consume carbs, they are broken down into glucose, which enters the bloodstream and boosts blood glucose levels. In reaction, the pancreas's beta cells secrete insulin. Insulin is released in proportion to the quantity of glucose in the blood, ensuring that blood glucose levels are controlled within a tight range.

Insulin's Mechanism of Action:

Insulin increases the absorption of glucose into cells by attaching to insulin receptors on the cell surface. This binding starts a cascade of events inside the cell that causes glucose transporters, particularly GLUT4, to migrate to the cell membrane and allow glucose to enter the cell. This mechanism is notably apparent in muscle and adipose tissue, where GLUT4 plays a key role in glucose uptake.

Regulation of Blood Glucose Levels:

Once inside the cells, glucose can be used immediately for energy through glycolysis or stored as glycogen in the liver and muscles. Insulin improves the storage of glucose by promoting glycogen synthesis (glycogenesis) and reducing the breakdown of glycogen (glycogenolysis). This guarantees that glucose is available for future energy needs.

Glucagon and Counter-Regulatory Mechanisms:

In contrast to insulin, glucagon is a hormone generated by the alpha cells of the pancreas that boosts blood glucose levels. When blood glucose levels fall too low, glucagon is released to encourage the breakdown of glycogen into glucose (glycogenolysis) and enhance the creation of glucose from non-carbohydrate sources (gluconeogenesis). This counter-regulatory mechanism guarantees that blood glucose levels do not drop dangerously low.

Insulin Resistance and Metabolic Disorders:

Insulin resistance occurs when cells become less sensitive to insulin, resulting in higher blood glucose levels. This disease generally precedes the development of type 2 diabetes. Insulin resistance can develop from several factors, including heredity, obesity, physical inactivity, and poor food. When insulin resistance occurs, the pancreas responds by manufacturing more insulin. Over time, this increasing demand can limit the pancreas's ability to generate sufficient insulin, leading to hyperglycemia and diabetes.

Management of Blood Glucose Levels:

Effective management of blood glucose levels needs a combination of food, exercise, and medication (if necessary). A balanced diet with an emphasis on low glycemic index foods can help regulate blood glucose levels. Regular physical exercise promotes insulin sensitivity, allowing the body to use glucose more effectively. In some circumstances, drugs such as metformin or insulin therapy may be required to maintain blood glucose control.

Understanding the role of insulin and the mechanisms of glucose regulation is critical for avoiding and managing metabolic diseases. Proper glucose management ensures that the body has a continuous supply of energy and lowers the risk of consequences linked with high or low blood glucose levels.

Caloric Impact: Addressing the Calorie Content of Sugar and Its Role in Our Diets

Sugars are a key source of calories in the human diet, giving fast energy but also contributing to excess calorie intake when ingested in excessive amounts. Understanding the caloric impact of sugar and its function in our meals is vital for maintaining a healthy balance.

Caloric Content of Sugar:

Sugars, including glucose, fructose, and sucrose, provide 4 calories per gram. This is similar to the caloric content of other carbohydrates. However, because sugars are commonly consumed in considerable quantities and are added to a wide range of meals and beverages, they can significantly contribute to overall calorie intake.

Sources of Dietary Sugar:

Dietary sugars come from both natural and supplemental sources. Natural sugars are present in fruits, vegetables, and dairy products. These foods also give critical elements such as vitamins, minerals, and fiber. Added sugars, on the other hand, are added to foods throughout processing and preparation. Common sources of added sugars include sodas, candy, cakes, cookies, and sweetened beverages. These foods frequently have little nutritional value beyond calories.

Impact on Total Calorie Intake:

Excessive consumption of added sugars can lead to an increase in total calorie intake, which can contribute to weight gain and obesity. This is particularly troubling because additional sugars produce "empty calories" that lack critical elements. High-calorie, sugar-rich foods can displace more healthy foods in the diet, leading to nutrient shortages.

Role of Sugar in Energy Balance:

Sugars are a rapid source of energy, making them ideal for acute energy needs, such as during severe physical exercise. However, because they are rapidly digested and absorbed, they might contribute to spikes and subsequent decreases in blood glucose levels, thereby triggering oscillations in energy levels and appetite.

Dietary Recommendations for Sugar Intake:

Health groups, like the American Heart Association (AHA) and the World Health Organization (WHO), advocate limiting added sugar intake to lower the risk of chronic diseases such as obesity, type 2 diabetes, and heart disease. The AHA proposes that women should restrict added sugar consumption to no more than 100 calories (approximately 25 grams or 6 teaspoons) per day, while men should limit intake to no more than 150 calories (about 37.5 grams or 9 teaspoons) per day.

Strategies for Reducing Sugar Intake:

To limit sugar intake and its accompanying caloric impact, try the following strategies:

Read Nutrition Labels: Check food labels for added sugars and choose items with low or no added sugar.

Limit Sugary Beverages: Reduce consumption of sodas, sweetened teas, and fruit drinks. Opt for water, unsweetened beverages, or liquids sweetened with natural fruit.

Choose entire Foods: Focus on entire fruits, vegetables, and whole grains, which give natural sugars along with fiber, vitamins, and minerals.

Modify dishes: When baking or cooking, lower the quantity of sugar in dishes and explore utilizing natural sweeteners like fruit puree or spices to provide taste without additional sugars.

By being cognizant of the caloric impact of sugar and making informed food choices, individuals can better regulate their calorie intake and support overall health and wellness.

Sweet Taste Perception: Unraveling the Mystery of Taste Buds and Sugar Cravings

The impression of sweetness is a complicated sensory experience impacted by taste buds, brain chemistry, and various psychological factors. Understanding how we experience sweetness and why we seek sugar can provide insight into the issues of limiting sugar consumption.

Taste Buds and Sweetness Perception:

Taste buds are sensory organs situated on the tongue, soft palate, and other areas of the mouth and throat. To each taste bud contains taste receptor cells that respond to five basic tastes: sweet, salty, sour, bitter, and umami.

When humans take sugar, it connects to special receptors on taste buds known as sweet taste receptors.

Sweet taste receptors are mostly made of two protein subunits: T1R2 and T1R3. These receptors are triggered when sugar molecules connect to them, providing signals to the brain that are perceived as sweetness. This activation occurs even with extremely little levels of sugar, explaining why we can detect sweetness even at low doses.

Brain Chemistry and Reward Pathways:

The experience of sweetness activates the brain's reward system, specifically the production of the neurotransmitter dopamine. Dopamine is related to pleasure and reward, giving a sensation of satisfaction when we ingest sweet foods. This reward response is similar to the action of several addictive substances, which is why sugar can be habit-forming and lead to cravings.

Psychological Factors Influencing Sugar Cravings:

Several psychological factors can influence sugar cravings and consumption patterns:

Emotional Eating: Many people resort to sweet meals for consolation during times of stress, melancholy, or boredom. This emotional eating can generate a positive feedback loop, increasing the relationship between sugar and emotional relief.

Learned Behaviors: Cultural and societal influences have a vital part in establishing our preferences for sweet meals. Celebrations, holidays, and social gatherings often involve sweet foods, reinforcing the relationship between sugar and happy experiences.

Marketing and Availability: The food business actively promotes sugary products, making them readily available and tempting. Attractive packaging, promotion, and smart placement in stores might boost the urge to purchase and consume sweet foods.

Biological Factors and Sweet Preferences:

Genetic and biological factors also contribute to individual variances in sweet taste perception and preferences. Some people may have a heightened sensitivity to sweetness, while others may require higher quantities of sugar to obtain the same level of happiness. Additionally, genetic variations in sweet taste receptors can alter how we perceive and appreciate sweet meals.

Managing Sugar Cravings:

Understanding the elements that generate sugar cravings can aid in establishing measures to manage them:

Balanced Diet: Eating a balanced diet that contains a variety of nutrients can help regulate blood sugar levels and lessen cravings for sweet foods. Ensuring enough intake of protein, fiber, and healthy fats can enhance satiety and lessen hunger.

Mindful Eating: Practicing mindful eating entails paying attention to hunger and fullness cues, relishing the flavor and texture of food, and avoiding distractions while eating. This can help prevent impulsive eating and improve awareness of sugar intake.

Healthy options: Replacing sugary snacks with healthier options can satisfy sweet cravings without the negative health implications. Fresh fruit, yogurt with a drizzle of honey, or almonds with a touch of dark chocolate can provide natural sweetness and nutritional benefits.

Stress Management: Finding non-food strategies to handle stress and emotions can lessen reliance on sugary comfort foods. Activities such as exercise, meditation, and indulging in hobbies can provide alternate sources of pleasure and relaxation.

The Role of Sweeteners:

Artificial and natural sweeteners offer alternatives to sugar that can help reduce calorie intake and control blood sugar levels. However, their use should be done with caution, as some sweeteners might have unforeseen health effects or contribute to sustaining a desire for extremely sweet foods.

Artificial Sweeteners: Common artificial sweeteners include aspartame, sucralose, and saccharin. These sweeteners are many times sweeter than sugar, allowing for fewer quantities to be utilized. They are typically found in diet sodas, sugar-free gum, and low-calorie foods. While they can help reduce calorie consumption, several studies reveal potential linkages to weight gain, metabolic problems, and changed gut microbiota.

Natural Sweeteners: Natural sweeteners including stevia, monk fruit extract, and erythritol offer a lower-calorie alternative to sugar. These sweeteners are sourced from plants and have a more favorable metabolic profile. However, they may still contribute to maintaining a predisposition for sweet tastes, and their long-term consequences on health require further research.

Understanding the complexity of sweet taste perception and sugar cravings can empower individuals to make informed choices about their sugar consumption. By studying the biological, psychological, and environmental aspects that influence sugar intake, it is feasible to establish techniques for regulating cravings and ensuring a balanced, healthful diet.

Chapter 2

The Origins of Sugar Consumption

The narrative of sugar consumption extends back thousands of years, with its roots profoundly ingrained in the evolution of human taste and agricultural methods. Sugar, in its original form, was likely ingested from naturally sweet sources such as fruits and honey. The need for sweetness is an integral element of the human palate, possibly emerging as a survival mechanism to detect energy-rich foods. The first cultivated sugar-producing plant was sugarcane, a tropical grass native to Southeast Asia.

Early Uses of Sugarcane:

Archaeological evidence shows that sugarcane was initially domesticated in New Guinea circa 8000 BCE. Early humans chewed the raw stalks to get the delicious nectar. As agricultural practices evolved, sugarcane growing extended across India and the neighboring regions. By 500 BCE, Indians had invented a process to crystallize sugar from cane juice, generating what we now know as granulated sugar. This breakthrough was a key turning point, changing sugar from a perishable liquid into a storable, transportable commodity.

The Spread of Sugar:

From India, the knowledge of sugar manufacturing went to Persia and the Islamic world. During the development of the Arab Empire in the 7th and 8th centuries, sugarcane cultivation and sugar production techniques were introduced to the Mediterranean, North Africa, and Spain. The Crusades also helped the spread of sugar as returning crusaders brought back knowledge and samples of this exotic sweetener.

Historical Context: The History of Sugar, From Ancient Times to Modern Day

Medieval Europe:

In medieval Europe, sugar was a costly luxury item, frequently referred to as "white gold." It was used sparingly in cooking and as a therapeutic element. The demand for sugar expanded steadily, but it remained a scarce and costly commodity due to restricted supply and the long, grueling trading routes required to transport it.

The Age of Exploration:

The Age of Exploration in the 15th and 16th centuries drastically transformed the sugar industry. European explorers, seeking new trade routes and profit, founded colonies in the Americas, where they found ideal conditions for sugarcane growth. The Caribbean, in particular, became a hub for sugar production, with islands such as Barbados, Jamaica, and Cuba becoming as important sugar producers.

The Atlantic Slave Trade:

The burgeoning sugar industry in the Americas had a bad side: it was primarily dependent on slave labor. The Atlantic slave trade forcefully carried millions of Africans to the New World to labor on sugar plantations. The conditions were severe, and the mortality rate among slaves was high. The transatlantic trade formed a triangle route: slaves from Africa were carried to the Americas, where they produced sugar and other items that were then sold to Europe.

Industrial Revolution:

The Industrial Revolution in the 18th and 19th centuries substantially altered the sugar sector. Advances in technology, like as steam-powered mills and improved refining processes, enhanced production efficiency and output. This century also witnessed the expansion of sugar beet agriculture in Europe, offering an alternate source of sugar that was less dependent on tropical conditions and colonial estates.

Modern Era:

In this era, sugar has become a pervasive part of the global diet. Advances in cultivation, processing, and transportation have made sugar widely available and affordable. However, the rise of processed meals and sugary beverages has led to greater consumption and associated health risks.

Cultural Significance: How Different Cultures Have Used and Perceived Sugar

Sugar has held a place of importance in numerous cultures, influencing culinary habits, religious ceremonies, and social norms. Its value extends beyond mere sweetness, touching into issues of identity, celebration, and tradition.

India: The Birthplace of Sugar:

In India, sugar has been vital to diet and culture for millennia. Traditional Indian sweets, known as mithai, are commonly produced with sugar and play a prominent part in festivals, religious events, and family gatherings.

Offerings of sweets are prevalent in Hindu rites, indicating prosperity and divine favor.

Middle East and Mediterranean:

In the Middle East and Mediterranean countries, sugar became a key element in confectionary and desserts. Influenced by Persian and Arab culinary traditions, these nations developed elaborate sweets such as baklava and Turkish delight, which remain popular today.

Europe: From Luxury to Commonplace:

In Europe, sugar changed from a luxury commodity to a staple ingredient. During the Renaissance, sugar was utilized in extravagant feasts and sugar sculptures, showcasing wealth and sophistication. By the 18th and 19th centuries, sugar had become more affordable, leading to the development of a rich heritage of pastries, cakes, and confections.

Americas: Cultural Fusion:

In the Americas, the mix of indigenous, African, and European culinary traditions developed a broad assortment of sweet delights. Sugarcane farming throughout the Caribbean and South America led to the development of items like rum and molasses. In North America, sugar became a significant ingredient in desserts such as pies, pastries, and candies, representing the melting pot of cultural influences.

Asia: Balancing Sweetness:

In many Asian cultures, the use of sugar is commonly harmonized with other flavors to create harmonious cuisine. In China, for example, sweet and sour flavors are regularly blended, whereas in Japan, the subtle sweetness of items like mochi and red bean paste is treasured.

Economic Impact: The Sugar Trade and Its Global Implications

The sugar trade has had major economic repercussions, shaping global trade networks, colonial economies, and modern markets.

Colonial Economies and the Triangular Trade:

During the colonial period, sugar production was a driving force behind the triangular trade. European nations created large sugar plantations in the Caribbean and South America, exploiting both the land and enslaved labor. The income gained from sugar production drove the rise of colonial economies and financed further expansion and exploitation.

Industrial Advancements:

The Industrial Revolution introduced technological improvements that transformed sugar production. Steam-powered mills, centrifugal machines for refining, and improved methods of extraction boosted efficiency and production. These advances enabled mass manufacturing and reduced costs, making sugar more available to a broader population.

Global Market Dynamics:

In the current era, the global sugar market is characterized by complicated trade dynamics. Major manufacturers include Brazil, India, China, and Thailand, each playing a key part in the global supply chain. International trade agreements, taxes, and subsidies influence the market, impacting prices and production practices.

Health and Economic Costs:

The ubiquitous availability and consumption of sugar have major health and economic effects. The rise in sugar-related health conditions, such as obesity, diabetes, and heart disease, places a major load on healthcare systems. Efforts to address these difficulties include public health campaigns, sugar tariffs, and laws on food labeling and advertising.

Sustainable Production and Fair Trade:

As knowledge of the environmental and social implications of sugar production rises, there is a growing focus on sustainable and ethical practices. Fairtrade programs attempt to ensure that producers receive fair compensation and that labor conditions fulfill ethical standards. Additionally, initiatives to lessen the environmental footprint of sugar production include sustainable agriculture practices, reduced water usage, and reduced chemical inputs.

The path of sugar from its ancient origins to its current global presence is a story of human inventiveness, cultural progress, and economic transformation. Understanding the historical context, cultural significance, and economic influence of sugar provides significant insights into its multifaceted function in society. By exploring these facets, we may better grasp the multidimensional nature of sugar and its influence on our lives.

Chapter 3

The Rise of Sugar Fear

The dread of sugar has become a prominent aspect of contemporary health discourse, driven by accumulating evidence of its potential effects and widespread media coverage. This anxiety over sugar is a relatively recent phenomenon, gaining pace in the late 20th and early 21st centuries. The modern diet, abundant in processed foods and sugary beverages, has heightened worries about sugar's role in several health disorders, including obesity, diabetes, and heart disease. This dread is generated by a combination of scientific study, media influence, and increasing government standards, all contributing to growing public knowledge and anxiety around sugar consumption.

Early Concerns: Initial Health Concerns and Scientific Studies on Sugar

Historical Context of Health Concerns:

Health worries concerning sugar are not entirely new. As early as the 18th century, medical practitioners hypothesized about the deleterious effects of excessive sugar consumption. However, these concerns were primarily anecdotal and lacked the empirical rigor required to affect public opinion or dietary choices considerably.

Post-War Changes and the Advent of Processed Foods:

The post-World War II era saw considerable changes in food trends, particularly in the United States and other industrialized nations. Advances in food processing technologies led to an increasing availability of inexpensive, calorie-dense, and sugar-laden items. During this period, sugar intake surged, leading to the first significant scientific inquiries into its health implications.

Pioneering Studies:

In the 1950s and 1960s, researchers began to study the potential health problems linked with high sugar intake. One of the earliest and most prominent investigations was undertaken by Dr. John Yudkin, a British physiologist and nutritionist. In his 1972 book "Pure, White, and Deadly," Yudkin contended that sugar was a primary cause of various chronic ailments, including heart disease and obesity. His findings met tremendous hostility from the sugar business and were initially disregarded by many in the scientific community.

Emergence of Evidence:

Despite early pushback, the body of research linking sugar to bad health consequences continues to rise. By the late 20th century, multiple studies had shown an association between high sugar consumption and an increased risk of obesity, type 2 diabetes, and cardiovascular disease. These discoveries sparked a reevaluation of sugar's place in the diet and fueled growing worries about its ubiquitous use in processed foods and beverages.

Media Influence: How Media Coverage Has Shaped Public Perception of Sugar

The Power of Media:

The media has played a major influence in molding the popular image of sugar. Sensational headlines, investigative documentaries, and high-profile publications have brought the risks of sugar to the forefront of public attention. This media coverage has enhanced scientific results and brought them to the attention of a broader audience.

Early Media Coverage:

In the 1970s and 1980s, media coverage of sugar was irregular and often lacked the depth needed to impact public opinion considerably. However, when more scientific information surfaced, media outlets began to take a deeper look at the potential effects of sugar. High-profile articles and investigative reports revealed the linkages between sugar consumption and chronic diseases, raising public interest and concern.

The Role of Documentaries and Books:

Documentaries and literature have been particularly effective in molding popular opinion of sugar. One notable example is the 2004 documentary "Super-Size Me," which, although mostly focused on fast food, also exposed the excessive sugar content in many processed goods. Another notable contribution came from journalist Gary Taubes, whose 2011 book "Why We Get Fat" and subsequent publications suggested that sugar, rather than fat, was a primary driver of obesity and other chronic diseases.

Social Media and Digital Influence:

The emergence of social media and internet platforms has further highlighted concerns about sugar. Health influencers, nutrition bloggers, and online communities have played a vital role in spreading information about the possible effects of sugar. Viral articles, infographics, and films have made difficult scientific results accessible to a large audience, adding to a growing public awareness and fear of sugar.

Impact of Celebrity Endorsements:

Celebrity endorsements and campaigning have also altered popular opinion of sugar. High-profile figures, including actresses, athletes, and health professionals, have spoken out about the risks of sugar and pushed sugar-free or low-sugar diets. Their endorsements have lent credence to the anti-sugar movement and prompted consumers to reevaluate their dietary choices.

Government Guidelines: Evolution of Dietary Guidelines Regarding Sugar

Early Dietary Recommendations:

Government dietary standards have altered greatly throughout the years, reflecting the growing understanding of sugar's role in health. In the early 20th century, dietary advice to focused primarily on ensuring enough nutrition and preventing deficiencies. Sugar was not considered a big worry, and its intake was typically encouraged as a source of instant energy.

Shifts in the Mid-20th Century:

In the mid-20th century, as the link between diet and chronic diseases became increasingly clear, dietary standards began to evolve. The 1977 Dietary Goals for the United States, established by the Senate Select Committee on Nutrition and Human Needs, marked a key turning point. The guidelines advocated limiting fat intake and ingesting more carbs, especially sweets, to lessen the risk of heart disease. This suggestion was later criticized for contributing to the growth in obesity and diabetes.

Emerging Evidence and Changing Guidelines:

As more evidence surfaced regarding the health dangers connected with sugar, government guidelines began to reflect growing concerns. The 1980 Dietary Guidelines for Americans, produced by the U.S. Department of Agriculture (USDA) and the Department of Health and Human Services (HHS), included advice to limit sugar intake for the first time. These rules have been modified every five years, with each iteration including new scientific results.

Recent Guidelines and Sugar Reduction:

In recent years, government recommendations have placed increased emphasis on limiting sugar consumption. The 2015-2020 Dietary Guidelines for Americans shown that added sugars contribute no more than 10% of daily caloric intake. This recommendation was based on studies linking high sugar intake to obesity, type 2 diabetes, and cardiovascular disease. The guidelines also underlined the necessity of reading food labels and choosing items with reduced sugar content.

International Efforts:

The concern about sugar is not restricted to the United States. International organizations and governments around the world have also made attempts to solve the issue. The World Health Organization (WHO) has issued guidelines proposing that added sugars make up less than 10% of total caloric intake, with a further decrease to below 5% for extra health advantages. Several countries have instituted sugar tariffs, rules on marketing sugary foods to children, and public health initiatives to curb sugar intake.

Public Health Campaigns and Education:

Public health campaigns and educational initiatives have played a vital role in converting government guidelines into effective advice for consumers. These activities aim to raise awareness about the consequences of excessive sugar consumption and provide practical advice for limiting sugar intake. Campaigns such as "Sugar Smart" in the UK and "Rethink Your Drink" in the US have worked to enlighten and empower individuals to make healthier dietary choices.

Chapter 4

Understanding Sugar

Sugar is a simple carbohydrate that occurs naturally in many foods and is sometimes added to foods for flavor and preservation. Chemically, sugars are classed as monosaccharides and disaccharides. Monosaccharides, the simplest form of sugar, comprise glucose, fructose, and galactose. Disaccharides are made of two monosaccharide molecules bound together and include sucrose (table sugar), lactose (milk sugar), and maltose (malt sugar). Understanding the different forms of sugars and their sources is vital for managing food intake and maintaining health.

Types of Sugar: Natural vs. Added Sugars and Their Sources

Natural Sugars:

Natural sugars are those found fundamentally in whole foods such as fruits, vegetables, dairy products, and some grains. These carbohydrates come with a package of critical elements like vitamins, minerals, fiber, and antioxidants, which contribute to general wellness. For instance, fructose is the principal sugar found in fruits, while lactose is the sugar contained in milk and dairy products.

Fruits: Contain fructose along with vitamins, fiber, and water, making them nutrient-dense options.

Vegetables: Some vegetables, like carrots and beets, have natural sugars that add to their nutritious worth.

Dairy Products: Milk and yogurt include lactose, which is helpful for energy and supplies calcium and protein.

Whole Grains: Whole grains provide tiny amounts of natural sugars along with fiber, vitamins, and minerals.

Added Sugars:

Added sugars refer to any sugars or caloric sweeteners that are added to foods or beverages throughout processing or preparation. These include sugars added when cooking at home, as well as those added during the production process. Added sugars offer energy but lack the added nutrients present in whole foods with natural sugars. Common sources of added sugars include:

Soft Drinks: High in added sugars, frequently in the form of high-fructose corn syrup.

Candy and Sweets: Contain high amounts of added sugars.

Baked Goods: Pastries, cakes, and cookies generally include significant levels of added sugars.

Sweetened Dairy Products: Flavored yogurts and sweetened milk products can contain additional sugars.

Processed Foods: Sauces, dressings, and ready-to-eat meals may include hidden added sugars.

Sugar in the Body: How the Body Processes Different Types of Sugar

The body processes sugars through many metabolic pathways that transform these carbohydrates into energy.

This process begins in the digestive system and continues in many tissues, particularly the liver and muscles.

Digestive Process:

When sugar is ingested, it is broken down into its simplest forms—glucose, fructose, and galactose—by digestive enzymes. For example, sucrose is divided into glucose and fructose by the enzyme sucrase. Lactose is broken down into glucose and galactose by lactase. These monosaccharides are then absorbed into the bloodstream through small intestine.

Glucose Metabolism:

Glucose is the principal source of energy for the body's cells. Once absorbed, it goes through the bloodstream and is delivered to cells throughout the body. Insulin, a hormone generated by the pancreas, stimulates the uptake of glucose into cells where it is used for energy production. Much glucose is stored as glycogen in the liver and muscles for later use. If glycogen stores are full, extra glucose is converted to fat and stored in adipose tissue.

Fructose Metabolism:

Fructose, unlike glucose, is predominantly processed in the liver. When fructose reaches the liver, it is turned into glucose, glycogen, or fat. High consumption of fructose, especially from added sugars like high-fructose corn syrup, might overwhelm the liver's capacity to handle it efficiently, leading to the creation of triglycerides, which are stored as fat. This can contribute to fatty liver disease and other metabolic problems.

Galactose Metabolism:

Galactose is metabolized in the liver where it is turned into glucose-1-phosphate, which then enters glycolysis— a metabolic route that transforms glucose into energy. This step ensures that galactose, like glucose, may be utilized for energy production.

Daily Consumption: Recommended Daily Intake and Actual Consumption Trends

Recommended Daily Intake:

Health organizations have set guidelines for the recommended daily intake of sugars to enhance health and prevent chronic diseases. The World Health Organization (WHO) recommends that added sugars should constitute less than 10% of total daily calorie consumption, with a further decrease to below 5% for extra health advantages. For an average adult, this corresponds to around 25 grams (6 teaspoons) of additional sugar each day.

The American Heart Association (AHA) sets more specific guidelines, proposing that women restrict their intake of added sugars to no more than 100 calories per day (about 25 grams or 6 teaspoons), while men limit their intake to no more than 150 calories per day (approximately 37.5 grams or 9 teaspoons).

Actual Consumption Trends:

Despite these recommendations, actual sugar consumption in many nations far exceeds the advised limits. In the United States, the average adult consumes roughly 77 grams of added sugar per day, comparable to 19 teaspoons—more than triple the recommended amount for women and double for men. This high intake is mostly caused by the consumption of sugary beverages, snacks, and processed foods.

Impact on Health:

Excessive sugar consumption is associated with several undesirable health effects, including obesity, type 2 diabetes, cardiovascular disease, and dental cavities. High sugar intake can lead to weight gain by delivering additional calories without the nutritional benefits provided in entire foods. Additionally, it can produce rises in blood glucose levels, raising the risk of insulin resistance and diabetes.

Efforts to Reduce Consumption:

Public health programs and regulatory measures aim to minimize sugar consumption and encourage healthy dietary habits. These efforts include:

Nutrition Labeling: Mandating clear labeling of added sugars on food and beverage goods to assist consumers make informed choices.

Sugar fees: Implementing fees on sugary beverages to discourage excessive consumption and create income for public health programs.

Public Awareness Campaigns: Educating the public about the health dangers connected with high sugar intake and promoting healthier alternatives.

Reformulation of Products: Encouraging food manufacturers to lower the sugar level in their products and provide healthier options.

Understanding the many forms of sugars, how they are digested in the body, and the recommended versus actual consumption trends is crucial for making informed dietary decisions. Natural sugars contained in whole foods come with necessary nutrients that support health, while added sugars contribute empty calories and raise the risk of chronic diseases. By sticking to prescribed recommendations and being conscious of sugar intake, individuals can better manage their health and well-being.

Chapter 5

Myths and Misconceptions

Sugar is one of the most controversial topics in nutrition, with various myths and misconceptions regarding its effects on health. These misunderstandings can lead to undue fear and confusion about sugar consumption. By addressing these fallacies, we can better grasp the real influence of sugar on our health and make informed dietary decisions.

Myth 1: All Sugars Are Bad

One common myth is that all sugars are fundamentally hazardous for health. In actuality, the body needs glucose, a simple sugar, as a key energy source. Glucose is necessary for brain function, muscular movement, and overall cellular metabolism. Natural sugars found in fruits, vegetables, and dairy products come with critical nutrients including vitamins, minerals, and fiber, which are helpful for health. It is the additional sugars in processed meals and sugary drinks that represent a health risk when ingested in excess.

Myth 2: Sugar Causes Hyperactivity in Children

Another prevalent fallacy is that sugar causes hyperactivity in youngsters. This view has been perpetuated by anecdotal evidence and cultural myths. However, scientific study does not support this claim. Studies have consistently shown that sugar intake does not lead to hyperactive behavior in children. Factors such as context, excitement, and expectations often have a more significant impact on reported hyperactivity than sugar consumption itself.

Myth 3: Sugar is as Addictive as Drugs

The idea that sugar is equally addictive as drugs like cocaine or heroin is a sensationalized claim that has gained momentum in recent years. While it's true that consuming sugar can trigger the brain's reward system, similar to addictive chemicals, the comparison is unnecessarily basic. Unlike drug addiction, which can lead to serious physical dependency and withdrawal symptoms, sugar cravings are often controlled and can be managed by balanced eating habits. The occasional craving for a sweet pleasure does not amount to a hazardous addiction.

Myth 4: Eliminating Sugar is Necessary for Good Health

Some health enthusiasts argue for the entire exclusion of sugar from the diet, believing it to be vital for optimal health. While lowering added sugar intake is helpful, it is neither practicable nor required to eliminate all sugars. Natural sugars in whole foods supply significant nutrients and should be eaten as part of a balanced diet. The idea is to reduce the consumption of added sugars and focus on nutrient-dense foods.

Sugar and Obesity: The Role of Sugar in Weight Gain and Obesity

The Caloric Impact of Sugar

Sugar is a substantial source of empty calories, meaning it delivers energy without any vital elements. Consuming high amounts of sugary foods and beverages can lead to an excess caloric intake, which, if not balanced by physical activity, results in weight gain. Sugary drinks are particularly problematic since they can add a large number of calories without providing a feeling of fullness, leading to overconsumption.

High-Fructose Corn Syrup and Obesity

High-fructose corn syrup (HFCS) is a prevalent sweetener in many processed foods and beverages. It has been linked to the obesity epidemic due to its ubiquity and potential effects on metabolism. HFCS contains both glucose and fructose, with fructose being digested differently than glucose. Excessive fructose intake can lead to increased fat formation in the liver, insulin resistance, and higher levels of triglycerides, all of which contribute to obesity and metabolic syndrome.

Sugar-Sweetened Beverages and Weight Gain

Research has established a clear link between the use of sugar-sweetened drinks (SSBs) and weight gain. SSBs, including sodas, fruit drinks, and energy drinks, are the main sources of added sugars in the diet. Regular use of these beverages is connected with increased body weight and a higher risk of obesity in both children and adults. The liquid form of these carbohydrates is easily absorbed, leading to surges in blood glucose and insulin levels, which can promote fat formation.

Impact on Hormonal Regulation

Sugar consumption can also impact hormonal regulation associated with appetite and satiety. High sugar intake can affect the balance of hormones like leptin and ghrelin, which regulate hunger. Leptin, known as the "satiety hormone," informs the brain when we are full. Excessive sugar intake can lead to leptin resistance, diminishing the brain's ability to identify when the body has had enough food. Ghrelin, the "hunger hormone," promotes appetite and can be changed by sugar consumption, leading to increased hunger and overeating.

Behavioral and Environmental Factors

Behavioral and environmental factors also have a crucial influence on the link between sugar and obesity. The availability and marketing of sugary foods and beverages, particularly to youngsters, lead to their excessive consumption. Cultural norms and social influences might stimulate the ingestion of sugary treats, especially in festive circumstances. Additionally, sedentary lifestyles and restricted availability of healthful meals worsen the influence of high sugar consumption on weight gain and obesity.

Diabetes Connection: Clarifying the Link Between Sugar and Diabetes

Understanding Diabetes

Diabetes is a chronic disorder defined by excessive levels of glucose in the blood due to the body's inability to make or efficiently use insulin. There are two primary varieties of diabetes: type 1, an autoimmune disorder where the body assaults insulin-producing cells in the pancreas, and type 2, which is more common and connected to lifestyle factors such as nutrition, obesity, and physical inactivity. While type 1 diabetes is not caused by sugar consumption, type 2 diabetes is commonly related to dietary choices, particularly excessive sugar intake.

Sugar and Insulin Resistance

Insulin resistance is a crucial component in the development of type 2 diabetes. It occurs when the body's cells become less receptive to insulin, the hormone responsible for regulating blood glucose levels. High sugar intake, particularly from fructose, can contribute to insulin resistance by encouraging fat storage in the liver and raising inflammation. Over time, insulin resistance leads to greater blood sugar levels and increased demand on the pancreas to generate more insulin, eventually leading to type 2 diabetes.

Role of Fructose in Diabetes

Fructose, a component of both sucrose and high-fructose corn syrup, has a unique metabolic pathway that can contribute to the development of diabetes. Unlike glucose, which is largely used by cells for energy, fructose is processed in the liver. Excessive fructose intake can lead to fatty liver, increased synthesis of triglycerides, and insulin resistance. These metabolic abnormalities are closely linked to the development of type 2 diabetes.

Impact of Sugar-Sweetened Beverages

The intake of sugar-sweetened beverages is closely connected with an elevated risk of type 2 diabetes. Studies have indicated that persons who eat one or more sugary drinks per day have a significantly higher chance of acquiring type 2 diabetes compared to those who rarely use similar beverages. The quick absorption of liquid sugars leads to surges in blood glucose and insulin levels, contributing to insulin resistance and pancreatic stress.

Glycemic Index and Glycemic Load

The glycemic index (GI) and glycemic load (GL) are metrics that indicate how quickly and how much food elevates blood glucose levels. Foods with a high GI induce quick rises in blood sugar, whereas those with a low GI result in slower, more steady increases. Sugary foods and drinks often have a high GI, leading to immediate and large increases in blood glucose and insulin levels. Managing dietary consumption to include more low-GI foods will assist in maintaining stable blood sugar levels and lower the risk of diabetes.

Public Health Recommendations

Public health groups, like the World Health Organization (WHO) and the American Diabetes Association (ADA), advocate minimizing the intake of added sugars to lower the risk of type 2 diabetes. These guidelines highlight the necessity of a balanced diet, regular physical activity, and maintaining a healthy weight. By following this guidance, individuals can dramatically lower their chance of acquiring diabetes and improve general health.

The Broader Implications

The myths and misconceptions surrounding sugar, its role in obesity, and its connection to diabetes underline the necessity of understanding the intricacies of sugar use. While sugar itself is not intrinsically evil, excessive intake, particularly of added sugars, can lead to major health repercussions. By dispelling myths, acknowledging the role of sugar in weight gain and metabolic health, and understanding its impact on diabetes, we can make better-informed choices about our diets and general well-being.

Understanding the complex relationship between sugar, obesity, and diabetes is vital for making informed dietary choices and optimizing health outcomes. By addressing myths and misconceptions, acknowledging the impact of sugar on weight gain, and establishing the link between sugar and diabetes, we may better regulate our sugar intake and lower the risk of chronic diseases. This method demands a balanced attitude, emphasizing moderation and the importance of a nutrient-dense diet to support general health and well-being.

Relationship Between Sugar Consumption and Obesity

Understanding the Connection

The association between sugar consumption and obesity is a serious concern in public health, as rising rates of obesity are often connected to increased intake of added sugars. This relationship is complex, encompassing not simply the quantity of sugar consumed but also how it affects metabolism and overall health.

Caloric Density and Weight Gain

Sugar, particularly in the form of added sugars and sugary beverages, leads to weight gain due to its high caloric density. A gram of sugar delivers around four calories. Consuming sugary meals and drinks might lead to an excessive consumption of calories without supplying important nutrients. These additional calories are not easily compensated by the body, leading to weight gain if they are not balanced by physical activity. Liquid sugars, present in sodas and sweetened beverages, are particularly dangerous since they do not generate a feeling of fullness, leading to overconsumption.

Effects on Fat Storage

High sugar intake can influence fat storage in the body. Consuming significant amounts of sugar can lead to elevated levels of insulin, a hormone that regulates blood sugar. Chronic elevated insulin levels can promote fat deposition, particularly in the abdominal area. This is because insulin not only helps cells absorb glucose but also encourages the storage of fat in adipose tissues. Excessive sugar consumption can thus lead to an accumulation of visceral fat, which is connected with several health problems, including cardiovascular disease and type 2 diabetes.

High-Fructose Corn Syrup (HFCS) and Obesity

High-fructose corn syrup (HFCS) is a prevalent sweetener in many processed foods and beverages. HFCS includes both glucose and fructose, with the latter being metabolized differently by the liver. Excessive fructose intake has been associated with increased fat formation in the liver, insulin resistance, and a higher risk of obesity. Studies have demonstrated that high-fructose diets can lead to considerable weight gain and increased fat deposition compared to diets with reduced fructose content.

Sugary Beverages and Weight Gain

The intake of sugary beverages is a well-documented element in the obesity pandemic. These drinks are a substantial source of added sugars and calories, although they do not deliver the same satiety as solid foods. This can lead to excessive caloric intake since individuals may consume additional calories above their real energy demands. Research indicates that lowering the intake of sugary beverages can lead to weight loss and improved metabolic health.

Impact on Appetite Regulation

Sugar intake can alter the body's normal hunger-regulating processes. High sugar consumption can change the levels of hormones that influence hunger and satiety. For example, higher sugar intake can lead to leptin resistance, when the brain becomes less sensitive to signals that indicate fullness. As a result, individuals may have increased hunger and a predisposition to overeat. Additionally, high-sugar diets might influence the synthesis of ghrelin, a hormone that promotes appetite, perhaps leading to frequent and excessive eating.

Role of Overall Diet and Lifestyle

Dietary Patterns and Weight Management

The association between sugar consumption and obesity is influenced by overall dietary patterns. A diet high in refined carbs, saturated fats, and added sugars, along with poor consumption of fruits, vegetables, and whole grains, can contribute to weight gain and obesity. Balancing macronutrients and focusing on nutrient-dense diets is vital for managing weight and improving health. Incorporating a range of foods, such as lean proteins, healthy fats, and complex carbohydrates, can help stabilize blood sugar levels and assist weight management.

Physical Activity

Regular physical activity plays a significant role in maintaining weight and counteracting the effects of excessive sugar consumption. Exercise helps to burn off excess calories, enhance insulin sensitivity, and regulate hunger. Incorporating both aerobic exercises, such as walking or cycling, and strength training can boost metabolic health and help weight control. Physical activity also helps to relieve stress, which might lead to overeating and weight gain.

Behavioral Factors

Behavioral variables have a crucial influence on managing sugar consumption and overall weight. Emotional eating, stress, and behavioral habits all influence dietary choices and contribute to excessive intake of sugary foods. Addressing these behaviors through measures such as mindful eating, stress management techniques, and seeking help for emotional eating can contribute to better weight control and general health

Environmental Influences

The environment also affects eating choices and lifestyle behaviors. The availability of healthful dietary options, access to recreational locations, and societal norms can all affect sugar consumption and physical activity levels. Creating supportive environments that encourage healthy eating and active lifestyles is vital for avoiding and controlling obesity. Policies that promote access to nutritious foods and opportunities for physical activity can have a favorable impact on public health.

Hyperactivity in Children: Debunking the Myth of Sugar-Induced Hyperactivity

Scientific Evidence

One of the most popular misunderstandings regarding sugar is that it causes hyperactivity in youngsters. This idea is popular among parents and educators, sometimes leading to advice to restrict sugar intake to control behavior. However, scientific research does not support the concept that sugar directly causes hyperactivity. Numerous studies have studied this notion and found no significant evidence relating sugar consumption to increased hyperactive behavior in youngsters.

Placebo Effect

One reason for the prevalence of this misconception may be the placebo effect. When parents or caregivers believe that sugar promotes hyperactivity, they may be more likely to see and interpret behavior as hyperactive after sugar ingestion. In controlled investigations when neither the subjects nor the researchers know which group is receiving sugar or a placebo, no significant difference in hyperactivity levels has been detected.

Influence of Other Factors

Behavioral changes that are attributed to sugar intake may be impacted by other causes. For example, sugar is commonly ingested in circumstances that are stimulating or exciting, such as birthday parties or joyous gatherings. The excitement and social contacts at these times may contribute to increased activity levels in youngsters rather than the sugar itself. Additionally, youngsters may consume sugar alongside other meals and liquids that contribute to their behavior.

Nutrition and Behavior

While sugar itself may not induce hyperactivity, overall nutrition and diet can influence behavior and cognitive performance. A balanced diet that includes important nutrients, such as omega-3 fatty acids, vitamins, and minerals, improves brain function and stable mood. Ensuring that children have a well-rounded diet with enough nutrients can assist support healthy behavior and cognitive development.

Guidance for Parents

For parents concerned about their children's conduct, focusing on a balanced diet and general lifestyle is more successful than merely managing sugar intake. Encouraging healthy dietary habits, supporting regular physical activity, and providing a supportive environment for emotional and social development can contribute to better conduct and well-being. It is also crucial for parents to set realistic expectations and understand that occasional treats are a normal part of childhood.

Research and Education

Continued study and education are vital for refuting myths and providing correct information regarding the effects of sugar on behavior. Educating parents, educators, and healthcare professionals about the scientific evidence can help minimize misconceptions and encourage evidence-based strategies for managing children's health and behavior.

Chapter 6

Debunking Common Myths

The field of nutrition is rife with myths and misconceptions, particularly those that pertain to the consumption of sugar. These misconceptions are frequently the result of inaccurate interpretations of statistics, out-of-date information, or sensationalized claims in the media. To gain a better grasp of the facts of sugar consumption and the effects it has on health, it is essential to dispel these myths.

Americans Consume More Sugar Than Ever.

The idea that people in the United States are consuming more sugar than they ever have before is one of the most widespread misconceptions. This idea has been fostered by warnings from health professionals that have been issued for decades, broad coverage in the media, and increased awareness of health conditions that are tied to sugar, such as obesity and diabetes. Although there was indeed a huge increase in the use of sugar during the 20th century, the trends that have emerged in recent years tell a difference.

There is a decrease in the amount of added sugar that is being consumed.

According to data collected over the past few years, the amount of added sugar consumed by Americans has decreased, which runs counter to the widespread notion. The National Health and Nutrition Examination Survey (NHANES) and the United States Department of Agriculture (USDA) both provide extensive data on dietary patterns, including the amount of sugar that people consume.

Trends Over the Decades

During the late 20th century, particularly during the 1970s and 1990s, there was a considerable increase in the use of added sugars. This period corresponded with the growth of processed meals and sugary beverages.

However, since the early 2000s, there has been a gradual but consistent drop in the intake of added sugars.

Key Data Points

According to NHANES statistics, the average daily intake of added sugars among Americans peaked in the late 1990s and early 2000s, reaching roughly 25 teaspoons per day.

Since then, there has been a dramatic drop. By 2018, the average daily intake of added sugars has reduced to roughly 17 teaspoons per day.

This drop is found across many age groups and demographics, suggesting a larger shift in dietary habits and increased awareness of sugar use.

Reasons for the Decline

Several factors contribute to this decline:

Increased Public Knowledge: Over the past two decades, public health efforts have effectively raised knowledge about the detrimental health implications of excessive sugar consumption. Educational activities and labeling reforms have helped customers make more informed decisions.

Policy Changes: Government regulations and policies, such as the installation of updated nutrition labels that highlight added sugars, have played a significant influence. Additionally, some towns and governments have put fees on sugary beverages, which has resulted in lower consumption.

Sector Adjustments: The food and beverage sector has responded to consumer demand for healthier options by decreasing the sugar content in numerous products. Reformulating recipes and giving lower-sugar alternatives has become more prevalent.

Health Trends: There is an increasing trend towards healthy diets and lifestyles. More people are adopting diets that stress whole foods and reduce processed foods, contributing to the decline in added sugar intake.

Explain the Current Recommendations

Despite the drop in sugar consumption, it remains necessary to understand and follow the current dietary standards to maintain a healthy diet and prevent sugar-related health issues.

Dietary Guidelines for Americans

The Dietary Guidelines for Americans (DGA), issued jointly by the U.S. Department of Health and Human Services (HHS) and the USDA, give science-based guidance on nutrition and health. These guidelines are updated every five years to reflect the latest research and dietary trends.

Added Sugar Recommendations

The 2020–2025 Dietary Guidelines for Americans propose reducing added sugars to less than 10% of total daily calories. This translates to:

For adults, this translates to around 200 calories or about 12 teaspoons (50 grams) of added sugars per day, based on a 2,000-calorie diet.

For children, the limit varies based on age and caloric needs, but the general suggestion is to restrict added sugar intake as much as possible.

Sources of Added Sugars

Understanding where added sugars come from is vital for limiting intake. Common sources include:

Sugary Beverages: Soft drinks, fruit drinks, sports drinks, energy drinks, and sweetened teas are substantial contributors.

Snacks & Sweets: Baked foods, sweets, ice creams, and sweetened yogurt generally include large amounts of added sugars.

Condiments and Sauces: Many condiments, including ketchup, barbecue sauce, and salad dressings, have added sugars.

Processed Foods: Many processed and packaged foods, especially those not normally associated with sweetness, may have added sugars for flavor enhancement.

While the illusion that Americans are consuming more sugar than ever prevails, the reality is that there has been a substantial drop in added sugar intake over the past two decades. This development is a result of greater public awareness, regulatory changes, industry adjustments, and trends towards healthier lifestyles. Understanding and sticking to the current dietary guidelines for added sugars is vital for preserving health and preventing sugar-related health concerns. By making informed choices and adopting practical measures, individuals can effectively regulate their sugar intake and enhance their overall well-being.

Myth 2: Sugar Is Addictive

The concept that sugar is addictive has acquired mainstream acceptance, with many equating it to substances like narcotics and alcohol. This hypothesis claims that sugar can hijack the brain's reward system, resulting in cravings, withdrawals, and obsessive consumption. While sugar can be highly appealing and induce overconsumption, characterizing it as addictive in the same manner as narcotics is an oversimplification that lacks scientific evidence.

Dispel the Notion of Sugar Addiction

Scientific Understanding of Addiction

To understand whether sugar is addictive, it is important to analyze the scientific criteria for addiction. True addiction is characterized by compulsive seeking and use of a substance despite severe effects, physical dependence, tolerance, and withdrawal symptoms. These conditions are often met by substances such as alcohol, nicotine, and narcotics.

In contrast, while sugar can contribute to overconsumption and cravings, it does not meet the strict criteria for addiction. Studies in humans have not shown the kind of neurochemical and behavioral alterations that are found with addictive medications. Unlike addictive substances, sugar does not generate substantial withdrawal symptoms or require increasing doses for the same effect.

Behavioral and Psychological Factors

The notion of sugar addiction is often confounded with behavioral and psychological issues. Cravings for sweet foods can be motivated by emotional eating, stress, and regular patterns rather than a true addiction. For example, individuals could gravitate to sweet snacks for consolation during times of stress or despair, forming a psychological attachment rather than a physical dependency.

Overeating vs. Addiction

It is crucial to distinguish between excess and addiction. Overeating sugar can lead to undesirable health outcomes like obesity and diabetes, but this is an issue of dietary patterns and self-control rather than an addiction. Food, particularly sugar, can be tremendously satisfying, but it does not generate the obsessive craving for more that characterizes addiction to drugs or alcohol.

Discuss Dopamine Response and Pleasure

Dopamine and the Brain's Reward System

Dopamine is a neurotransmitter that plays a major part in the brain's reward system. It is released in reaction to enjoyable activities, like feeding, which promotes behaviors important for survival. When we consume sugar, dopamine is released, providing a feeling of pleasure and fulfillment.

Comparison to Addictive Substances

While sugar consumption triggers dopamine release, it is not unique in this sense. Many activities, such as social contact, exercise, and various sorts of food, also release dopamine. The key variation is in the intensity and pattern of dopamine release. Addictive chemicals generate a considerably more massive and persistent release of dopamine, leading to the highly reinforcing and compulsive behavior seen in addiction.

The Pleasure of Eating Sugar

The pleasurable response to sugar is a natural feature of human biology, meant to encourage the ingestion of energy-dense foods in times of scarcity. However, in modern civilizations with sufficient food supply, this natural desire can lead to overconsumption. This is not equivalent to addiction but shows the need for mindful eating and moderation.

Neuroscientific Research

Neuroscientific research demonstrates that while sugar can activate the brain's reward centers, the response is not as powerful or detrimental as that induced by addictive narcotics. Studies employing brain imaging techniques like fMRI have demonstrated that while there is increased activity in response to sugar, it is similar to reactions seen with other pleasurable experiences and does not imply addiction.

Myth 3: White Sugar Is Bleached

Another prevalent misunderstanding is that white sugar is bleached to attain its pure hue, leading to concerns about chemical residues and safety. This fallacy likely originates from misunderstandings about the sugar refining process and the vocabulary used to describe it.

The Refining Process of White Sugar

White sugar is obtained from sugarcane or sugar beets. The refining process involves multiple processes to remove contaminants and generate the final product. Here's a simple summary of how white sugar is made:

Extraction: Sugarcane or sugar beets are collected and processed to extract the juice. This juice contains a blend of water, sugars, and plant components.

Clarification: The extracted juice is boiled and treated with lime (calcium hydroxide) to neutralize acids and eliminate contaminants. This procedure helps to clarify the juice by causing contaminants to coagulate and be filtered away.

Evaporation: The clarified juice is next heated to evaporate water, resulting in a thick syrup known as raw sugar.

Crystallization: The syrup is further concentrated by boiling, leading to the creation of sugar crystals. These crystals are removed from the remaining liquid (molasses) using centrifuges.

Refining: The raw sugar crystals are dissolved in water and filtered through activated carbon or bone char to eliminate remaining impurities and color. This procedure does not use bleaching agents but relies on physical filtration.

Final Crystallization: The filtered solution is heated again to crystallize the sugar, which is then dried and packed as white sugar.

Clarifying the Misconception

The term "bleaching" sometimes conjures thoughts of harsh chemicals, but in the context of sugar refining, it refers to the removal of color and impurities by physical filtration procedures. No chlorine bleach or comparable chemicals are utilized. Instead, natural decolorizing chemicals like activated carbon are applied to produce the necessary purity and whiteness.

Safety and Quality Assurance

The sugar refining process is subject to strong quality control and safety regulations to guarantee that the finished product is safe for consumption. Regulatory authorities like the Food and Drug Administration (FDA) regulate these processes, ensuring that white sugar is free from hazardous residues and meets purity criteria.

Comparing White Sugar to Other Sugars

While white sugar is the most refined form, other varieties of sugar, including brown sugar and raw sugar, undergo fewer refining stages and retain more of the natural molasses component. The decision between these sugars frequently comes down to personal preference and culinary use, rather than significant distinctions in health impact.

Describe the Natural Process of Sugar Production

Sugar production is a fascinating and sophisticated process that has evolved over the ages. It begins with the production of sugarcane or sugar beets, two key sources of sugar. Each plant performs a series of procedures to extract and refine the sweet crystalline component known as sucrose.

Sugarcane Cultivation and Harvesting

Sugarcane is a tropical grass that demands warm conditions and adequate water. It is typically farmed in nations like Brazil, India, and Thailand. The cultivation procedure involves planting sugarcane stalks, which grow into tall, jointed stems. These stems are rich in sucrose, which can be extracted for sugar manufacture.

Once mature, the sugarcane is harvested, usually by cutting the stalks close to the ground. Harvesting can be done manually or using mechanical harvesters, depending on the amount of production and available technology. The gathered sugarcane is transported to mills for processing.

Sugar Beet Cultivation and Harvesting

Sugar beets are grown in temperate areas and are largely produced in regions like Europe, North America, and Russia. Unlike sugarcane, sugar beets are root crops. They are cultivated in fields and require correct soil preparation, fertilizer, and watering.

When the sugar beets reach maturity, they are harvested using technology that lifts the beets from the earth. The beets are then washed to eliminate dirt and debris before being sent to processing facilities.

Extraction of Sugar

The extraction process for both sugarcane and sugar beets contain several important steps:

Juice Extraction: The harvested sugar cane is crushed in mills to extract the juice. For sugar beets, the roots are sliced into thin strips called cassettes and then steeped in boiling water to extract the juice.

Juice Clarification: The extracted juice contains contaminants, including plant fibers, soil, and other organic debris. To clear the juice, it is boiled and treated with lime (calcium hydroxide) to neutralize acids and coagulate contaminants. This results in a clearer juice that can be further processed.

Evaporation: The cleared juice is next heated to evaporate water, resulting in a thick syrup known as raw sugar juice. This process concentrates the sugar concentration and prepares the juice for crystallization.

Crystallization: The concentrated syrup is seeded with small sugar crystals to induce crystallization. As the syrup cools, sucrose crystals form and expand. These crystals are removed from the remaining liquid, or molasses, using centrifuges.

Explain How White Sugar Is Obtained

The manufacturing of white sugar needs additional refining stages to ensure the purity and consistency of the finished product. This refining process removes any leftover impurities and color, resulting in the typical white granules used in kitchens worldwide.

Refining Raw Sugar

The raw sugar crystals obtained from the initial extraction procedure contain molasses and other impurities that give them a dark tint. To generate white sugar, these raw crystals undergo further refining:

Dissolution: The raw sugar is dissolved in water to make a syrup. This procedure helps to separate the sugar from non-sugar components.

Filtration: The syrup is filtered to remove insoluble contaminants. Activated carbon or bone char is commonly used in this process to decolorize the syrup and eliminate any remaining molasses. It is vital to note that no bleaching agents are employed; the color is removed by physical filtration.

Evaporation and Crystallization: The purified syrup is cooked again to concentrate the sugar content. This concentrated syrup is then seeded with sugar crystals to induce crystallization. As the syrup cools, pure white sugar crystals develop.

Centrifugation: The sugar crystals are separated from the remaining liquid using centrifuges. This process guarantees that the crystals are free from any lingering contaminants or color.

Drying and Packaging: The white sugar crystals are dried to remove any leftover moisture. The completed product is then packaged and ready for distribution and consumption.

Myth 4: "Reduced Sugar" Means Fewer Calories

The word "reduced sugar" on product labels can be misleading for consumers who are seeking to regulate their calorie consumption. Many consumers assume that items labeled as "reduced sugar" are also lower in calories, however, this is not necessarily the case. Understanding the complexities underlying this labeling will help consumers make more educated choices.

What Does "Reduced Sugar" Mean?

According to food labeling standards, "reduced sugar" signifies that the product has at least 25% less sugar than the regular version of the same product. However, this reduction in sugar does not necessarily equal a significant reduction in calories.

Caloric Content and Sugar Replacements

To maintain the taste and texture of the original product, manufacturers often replace the missing sugar with other components. These alternatives can include artificial sweeteners, sugar alcohols, or additional lipids and carbs. While artificial sweeteners and sugar alcohols may contribute fewer or no calories, additional fats and carbohydrates can maintain or even increase the overall calorie load.

Understanding the Ingredients

When analyzing "reduced sugar" products, it is vital to examine the ingredient list and nutritional facts. Look for extra additives like maltodextrin, a carbohydrate that can boost calorie count or fats that are used to preserve the product's texture. These additions can counteract the calorie reduction predicted by lower sugar content.

Consumer Misconceptions

The misperception that "reduced sugar" means fewer calories might lead to inadvertent overconsumption. Believing they are picking a healthier option, consumers might eat more of the reduced-sugar food, resulting in an equal or larger calorie intake compared to the standard form.

Case Study: Reduced-Sugar Products

Consider a popular reduced-sugar peanut butter. The normal version contains 190 calories and 3 grams of sugar per serving. The reduced-sugar version consist of 180 calories and 1 gram of sugar per serving. While the sugar content is lower, the calorie difference is minimal. Consumers focusing primarily on sugar reduction can ignore the reality that they are not considerably reducing their overall caloric intake.

Regulatory Standards and Labeling

Food labeling standards are supposed to provide customers with critical information, yet they can occasionally generate misunderstanding. The term "reduced sugar" is regulated, although its application needs careful assessment of the total nutritional profile. Consumers should be aware that sugar reduction does not inherently guarantee a healthier product if other ingredients compensate for the reduced sugar.

Uncover the Truth Behind Reduced-Sugar Products

Marketing Tactics

Food makers are aware of the increased desire for healthier products and often utilize "reduced sugar" as a marketing technique. Packaging may promote the lower sugar level conspicuously, deflecting attention from other nutritional elements such as calorie count, fat content, or the inclusion of artificial additives.

Artificial Sweeteners and Health Considerations

Many reduced-sugar goods incorporate artificial sweeteners like aspartame, sucralose, or stevia. While artificial sweeteners can reduce calorie intake, their health implications are a topic of ongoing dispute. Some research implies potential linkages to metabolic alterations, digestive difficulties, or altered gut microbiota. Consumers should consider these criteria while buying reduced-sugar goods.

Balancing Sugar Reduction with Overall Nutrition

A holistic approach to diet requires going beyond just sugar content. It is crucial to consider the complete nutritional profile of a product, including calories, fats, proteins, fiber, and vitamins. A product may have lower sugar but still, be heavy in harmful fats or poor in critical nutrients.

Practical Tips for Consumers

Read Labels Carefully: Look beyond marketing claims and analyze the full ingredient list and nutritional information.

Examine Products: When deciding between regular and reduced-sugar versions, examine the overall nutritional composition, including calories, fats, and other substances.

Mindful Eating: Be aware of portion sizes and total consumption. Reduced sugar does not mean you may eat more without consequences.

Focus on Whole Foods: Incorporate more whole foods like fruits, vegetables, and whole grains into your diet. These foods naturally contain less added sugar and provide critical nutrients.

Be Skeptical of Claims: Understand that "reduced sugar" is simply one facet of a product's nutritional

profile. Consider the product's healthfulness in its
totality.

Compare Nutrient Packages

When picking foods, it's vital to compare nutrient
packages to grasp the overall nutritional value of what
we consume. Different foods, even those with
comparable calorie counts or sugar concentrations, might
give radically different advantages in terms of vitamins,
minerals, fiber, and other critical nutrients.

Whole Foods vs. Processed Foods

Whole foods, such as fruits, vegetables, whole grains,
nuts, and seeds, are nutrient-dense, meaning they supply
a high number of vitamins, minerals, and other beneficial
elements relative to their calorie content. These foods are
minimally processed and free from added sugars,
harmful fats, and artificial additives. For example, an
apple not only delivers natural sugars but also gives
fiber, vitamin C, and antioxidants.

In contrast, processed foods often have additional sugars
and fats that enhance flavor and shelf life but offer

little nutritional value. A candy bar could have the same calorie count as an apple but lacks the fiber, vitamins, and minerals, delivering instead empty calories that can contribute to weight gain and health risks if consumed in excess.

Nutrient Density

Nutrient density refers to the sum of nutrients a food supplies about the calories it contains. Foods like leafy greens, berries, and lean proteins are considered nutrient-dense. They improve general health and well-being by giving critical nutrients without excessive calories. In contrast, sugary snacks and beverages are calorie-dense but nutrient-poor, giving energy without major health advantages.

Micronutrient Comparison

Comparing nutrient packages also involves looking at the micronutrient composition, including vitamins and minerals. For instance, a serving of fortified morning cereal might provide considerable amounts of B vitamins, iron, and calcium thanks to fortification.

However, it could also include high levels of added sugars and low fiber. On the other hand, a bowl of oatmeal with fresh fruit delivers natural supplies of fiber, vitamins, and minerals without added sugars.

Reading Labels

Understanding food labels is vital for comparing nutrient packages. Look for:

Serving Size: Ensure you're comparing identical serving sizes.

Calories: Consider the energy delivered per serving.

Total Sugars and Added Sugars: Differentiate between naturally occurring sugars and those added during processing.

Fiber: Higher fiber content often implies a healthier choice.

Vitamins and Minerals: Check for critical nutrients like vitamin A, vitamin C, calcium, and iron.

Ingredients List: The shorter and more identifiable the component list, the better.

Myth 5: Sugar Causes Chronic Diseases

One of the most common misunderstandings regarding sugar is that it directly causes chronic diseases such as obesity, diabetes, and heart disease. While high sugar intake might contribute to health concerns, it is extremely simplistic and inaccurate to imply that sugar alone is the culprit.

Obesity

Obesity is a complex disorder influenced by various variables, including genetics, lifestyle, and cuisine. While high sugar intake can contribute to weight gain, especially from sugary beverages and snacks, it is not the main cause. Total calorie consumption, physical activity levels, and overall dietary patterns play major impacts. Diets high in added sugars generally correspond with low nutrient density, leading to weight gain and metabolic difficulties when consumed in excess.

Diabetes

The association between sugar and diabetes, particularly type 2 diabetes, is widely misinterpreted. Type 2 diabetes is characterized by insulin resistance when the body's cells do not respond adequately to insulin. While high sugar intake can lead to weight gain and a higher risk of developing type 2 diabetes, it is not the sole reason. Genetics, lack of physical activity, and other dietary components, such as processed carbs and harmful fats, also contribute to the development of diabetes.

Heart Disease

Heart disease is influenced by a range of factors, including high blood pressure, excessive cholesterol, smoking, and lack of exercise. Diets high in added sugars can contribute to heart disease by increasing calorie consumption, leading to obesity, and changing blood lipid levels. However, it is vital to evaluate the total diet. Saturated fats, trans fats, and high sodium intake are also significant contributors to heart disease. A balanced diet that contains healthy fats, fiber, and nutrient-dense foods is vital for heart health.

Address the Link Between Sugar and Obesity, Diabetes, and heart disease

Obesity

The association between sugar and obesity is mostly related to the consumption of sugary beverages and high-calorie foods. These things can lead to an excessive calorie intake because they are commonly consumed in addition to normal meals. Sugary drinks like sodas and fruit juices are particularly harmful since they give liquid calories that do not contribute to satiety, leading to increased overall calorie consumption. However, obesity develops from a complicated interaction of factors, including overall calorie intake, physical inactivity, genetic susceptibility, and socioeconomic circumstances.

Diabetes

The link between sugar and diabetes is commonly stressed in talks about nutrition and health. While high sugar intake can contribute to weight gain and increase the risk of type 2 diabetes, it is not the primary cause. Type 2 diabetes is a complex illness impacted by genetic and lifestyle factors. Consuming a balanced diet, maintaining a healthy weight, and engaging in regular physical activity are crucial in preventing diabetes. It's vital to clarify between type 1 and type 2 diabetes, as type 1 diabetes is an autoimmune disorder not linked to sugar intake.

Heart Disease

Excessive sugar consumption can damage heart health in numerous ways. Diets heavy in added sugars can lead to obesity, which is a risk factor for heart disease. High sugar intake can also elevate blood pressure and increase inflammation, both of which are associated with cardiovascular disease. Additionally, consuming too much sugar can lead to greater triglyceride levels and decreased levels of HDL (good) cholesterol, further raising the risk of heart disease. However, it is vital to evaluate the whole diet and lifestyle. A diet high in fruits, vegetables, whole grains, and healthy fats, together with regular exercise, is helpful for heart health.

Balanced Perspective

Addressing the link between sugar and chronic diseases demands a balanced perspective. While it is vital to minimize added sugar intake, focusing simply on sugar ignores other critical dietary and lifestyle aspects. A holistic approach to health analyzes total calorie consumption, nutrient density, physical exercise, and general lifestyle behaviors. Encouraging balanced diets rich in whole foods and supporting active lifestyles are crucial measures in preventing and managing chronic diseases.

knowing the intricacies of sugar consumption and its consequences on health is crucial. While beliefs regarding sugar and chronic diseases linger, it is vital to look at the wider picture. Sugar, when ingested in moderation as part of a balanced diet, does not necessarily induce chronic diseases. However, excessive intake, particularly from sugary beverages and processed meals, might contribute to health concerns. Educating people about the complete nutritional profile of foods, promoting balanced meals, and encouraging active lives are vital to improving public health and refuting prevalent beliefs regarding sugar.

Chapter 7

The Real Health Impacts of Sugar

Sugar, a widespread component of the modern diet, has a wide range of consequences on health. Understanding these effects needs a thorough look at both the short-term and long-term repercussions of sugar consumption. While sugar is a natural source of energy, excessive ingestion can lead to different health complications, some of which are immediate, while others manifest over time.

Short-term Effects: Immediate Effects of Sugar on the Body

When you take sugar, the body experiences instant consequences that can be both useful and negative, depending on the context and quantity consumed.

Energy Boost and Mood Elevation

One of the most prominent short-term consequences of sugar is its capacity to give a quick supply of energy. Simple carbohydrates like glucose are easily absorbed into the system, increasing blood sugar levels. This can result in an immediate energy boost and mood elevation, which is why many people reach for sugary snacks or drinks when they feel sleepy or sluggish.

Blood Sugar Spikes and Crashes

However, this rapid absorption also leads to a sudden rise in blood sugar levels, followed by an equally rapid decline. This sequence of spikes and crashes can make variations in energy levels and mood. After the first high, people often experience a "sugar crash," marked by feelings of weariness, irritation, and hunger. These oscillations can be particularly severe in patients with insulin resistance or other metabolic problems.

Impact on Cognitive Function

Short-term sugar consumption can potentially impact cognitive performance. Some studies suggest that moderate sugar intake can temporarily improve mental performance and memory due to the increased availability of glucose to the brain. However, excessive sugar intake, particularly from sugary drinks and snacks, has been associated with poorer cognitive performance and decreased alertness, perhaps due to the ensuing energy crash and potential inflammatory effects on the brain.

Dental Health

The immediate consequences of sugar on dental health are very considerable. Sugar provides a food source for bacteria in the mouth, which creates acid as a consequence of sugar metabolism. This acid can dissolve tooth enamel, leading to cavities and tooth rot. Maintaining proper oral hygiene and controlling sugar intake is vital for preventing these instant harmful impacts on tooth health.

Long-term Consequences: Chronic Diseases Linked to Excessive Sugar Consumption

While the short-term effects of sugar are typically reversible and tolerable, the long-term implications of excessive sugar consumption are significantly more harmful and can lead to chronic disorders.

Obesity

One of the most well-documented long-term impacts of excessive sugar consumption is obesity. High sugar intake, particularly from sugary beverages and processed foods, adds to an increased caloric intake without delivering any nutritional benefits. Over time, this can lead to weight gain and obesity, which are risk factors for a range of other health concerns, including type 2 diabetes, cardiovascular disease, and some malignancies.

Insulin Resistance and Type 2 Diabetes

Chronic overconsumption of sugar can lead to insulin resistance, a disease where the body's cells become less receptive to insulin. Insulin is a hormone that helps regulate blood sugar levels by facilitating the uptake of glucose into cells. When cells grow resistant to insulin, blood sugar levels keep on elevated, leading to type 2 diabetes. This syndrome increases the risk of various problems, including neuropathy, kidney impairment, and cardiovascular disease.

Cardiovascular Disease

Excessive sugar intake is also linked to cardiovascular disease. High sugar consumption can lead to increased triglyceride levels, lower HDL (good) cholesterol levels, and higher LDL (bad) cholesterol levels, all of which are risk factors for heart disease. Additionally, obesity and type 2 diabetes, both associated with high sugar intake, significantly enhance the chance of having cardiovascular problems. Chronic inflammation, another result of high sugar intake, is also a crucial contributor to the development of atherosclerosis and other heart problems.

Non-Alcoholic Fatty Liver Disease (NAFLD)

Another significant long-term consequence of increased sugar intake is non-alcoholic fatty liver disease (NAFLD). This illness is considered by the buildup of fat in the liver, which can progress to hepatic inflammation, fibrosis, and eventually cirrhosis. Fructose, a component of sugar, is metabolized largely by the liver and can contribute to the development of NAFLD when ingested in excess, particularly in the form of high-fructose corn syrup present in many processed foods and beverages.

Links Between Sugar Consumption and Conditions Like Diabetes, Heart Disease, and Cancer

Diabetes

The association between sugar consumption and diabetes is complicated. While sugar alone does not directly cause diabetes, high ingestion can lead to circumstances that raise the chance of developing type 2 diabetes. The major mechanism includes insulin resistance, which can develop from chronic excessive sugar intake, particularly from sugary beverages that contribute to rapid spikes in blood glucose and insulin levels. Over time, this can exhaust the insulin-producing cells of the pancreas, leading to decreased insulin production and the establishment of type 2 diabetes.

Heart Disease

High sugar consumption contributes to heart disease through multiple routes. Firstly, it leads to obesity, a major risk factor for cardiovascular problems. Secondly, high sugar intake increases triglyceride levels, which can cause atherosclerosis, the accumulation of fatty deposits in the arteries. This disorder inhibits blood flow and can result in heart attacks and strokes. Additionally, high-sugar diets are correlated to elevated blood pressure and inflammation, all of which contribute to the development of heart disease.

Cancer

There is mounting evidence associating high sugar consumption with an increased risk of some malignancies. Obesity, driven by excessive sugar intake, is a well-known risk factor for numerous types of cancer, including breast, colorectal, and pancreatic cancers. heavy insulin levels and insulin resistance, typical in individuals with heavy sugar diets, can also stimulate cancer cell proliferation. Insulin and insulin-like growth factor (IGF) can boost cell proliferation and block apoptosis (programmed cell death), generating an environment conducive to cancer formation.

Furthermore, chronic inflammation, another consequence of high sugar intake, is a recognized component in the development of cancer. Inflammatory processes can lead to DNA damage and the genesis and growth of malignant cells. While additional research is needed to completely understand the precise processes linking sugar to cancer, the present evidence suggests that restricting sugar intake can reduce the incidence of obesity-related malignancies and improve general health.

Explain the Impact of Sugar on Blood Glucose Levels

Sugar, particularly in the form of glucose, has a direct and immediate impact on blood glucose levels. When you consume foods containing sugar, your digestive system breaks down these sugars into glucose, which subsequently enters the circulation. This process boosts blood glucose levels and prompts several physiological reactions to preserve balance.

Rapid Increase in Blood Glucose

Upon consuming sugar, especially simple carbohydrates like table sugar (sucrose), blood glucose levels rise rapidly. This is because simple carbohydrates are readily digested and absorbed into the bloodstream. The glycemic index (GI) of a food assesses how quickly it raises blood glucose levels; items with high GI values, such as sugary drinks and candy, induce sharp spikes in blood glucose.

Insulin Response

In response to the rise in blood glucose, the pancreas secretes insulin, a hormone that stimulates the uptake of glucose by cells, where it can be utilized for energy or stored as glycogen in the liver and muscles. Insulin effectively decreases blood glucose levels by allowing cells to absorb glucose, reducing hyperglycemia (high blood sugar levels).

Blood Glucose Regulation

Maintaining blood glucose levels within a restricted range is vital for general health. Persistent high blood glucose levels can develop into insulin resistance when cells become less receptive to insulin. This syndrome can lead to type 2 diabetes if not controlled. Conversely, too much insulin can produce hypoglycemia (low blood sugar levels), leading to symptoms like dizziness, confusion, and fainting.

Factors Affecting Blood Glucose Response

Several factors determine how the body responds to sugar intake. These include the type of sugar consumed, the presence of other nutrients (including fiber, fat, and protein), and individual metabolic variables. For example, diets high in fiber slow down the digestion and absorption of sugar, resulting in a more gradual rise in blood glucose levels. On the other hand, sugary beverages ingested on an empty stomach might induce quick surges.

Dental Health: Discuss Sugar's Role in Tooth Decay

The association between sugar and dental health is well-established, with sugar being the main cause of the development of tooth decay. Tooth decay, commonly known as dental caries or cavities, occurs when the hard surface of the teeth is attacked by acids produced by bacteria in the mouth.

Sugar is a Food Source for Bacteria

Sugar serves as a food supply for bacteria in the mouth, particularly Streptococcus mutans and Lactobacillus species. When these bacteria metabolize sugar, they produce acids as a byproduct. These acids can

demineralize and tear down the enamel, the hard outer
coating of the tooth, which can lead to cavities.

Formation of Plaque

Plaque is a sticky, white film of bacteria and
carbohydrates that builds on the teeth. When you ingest
sugary foods and beverages, the bacteria in plaque turn
the sugars into acid. If plaque is not eliminated
consistently through brushing and flossing, the acid can
destroy tooth enamel and create cavities.

Acidic Environment and Enamel Erosion

The acids produced by bacterial breakdown of sugar
reduce the pH in the mouth, creating an acidic
environment. Tooth enamel begins to demineralize and
lose its structure when the pH dips below 5.5. Repeated
exposure to acid attacks without appropriate time for
remineralization can lead to the progressive degradation
of enamel and the creation of cavities.

Types of Sugary Foods and Their Impact

Not all sweet foods have the same impact on tooth health. Sticky and chewy sweets, like caramels and gummy candies, tend to stay on teeth for longer periods, providing a persistent food source for bacteria and raising the risk of dental decay. Sugary drinks, such as sodas and fruit juices, also offer a substantial risk because they can coat the teeth with sugar and acid.

Prevention and Treatment Strategies

Preventing and treating the detrimental effects of sugar on blood glucose levels and tooth health needs a mix of dietary management, proper oral hygiene, and frequent healthcare practices.

Dietary Management

Limit Sugar Intake: Reducing the consumption of added sugars is vital. This can be achieved by eliminating sugary drinks, candy, and processed foods rich in sugar. Opt for entire meals like fruits, vegetables, and whole grains, which have a lower glycemic index and include critical minerals and fiber.

Balanced Diet: A diet rich in fiber, healthy fats, and proteins helps control blood glucose levels by slowing down the absorption of sugar. Including foods with low glycemic indices, such as legumes and nuts, can minimize rapid rises in blood sugar.

Hydration: Drinking plenty of water helps wash away food particles and sugars from the mouth, minimalizing the risk of tooth decay. Water also aids in maintaining hydration and improves general metabolic functioning.

Oral Hygiene Practices

Regular Brushing and Flossing: Brushing teeth at least twice a day with fluoride toothpaste and flossing every day are vital routines for removing plaque and preventing cavities. Fluoride reinforces tooth enamel, making it more resistant to acid attacks.

Dental exams: Regular dental appointments for expert cleanings and exams help spot early symptoms of tooth decay and other oral health issues. Dentists can administer fluoride treatments and sealants to safeguard teeth.

Mouthwash: Using an antibiotic mouthwash can help lower bacterial load in the mouth and lessen the incidence of cavities and gum disease.

Medical Interventions

Insulin Therapy: For persons with diabetes or insulin resistance, maintaining blood glucose levels using insulin therapy and medicines is critical. Regular monitoring of blood glucose levels helps change treatment regimens and prevent problems.

Dental Treatments: For existing cavities, dental fillings, crowns, and other restorative treatments are necessary to heal tooth damage. Advanced cases of tooth decay may necessitate more extensive procedures like root canals or extractions.

Lifestyle Modifications

Regular Exercise: Physical activity helps enhance insulin sensitivity and manage blood glucose levels. Exercise also promotes general cardiovascular health and weight management.

Stress Management: Chronic stress can impair blood glucose regulation and contribute to unhealthy eating behaviors. Practices like meditation, yoga, and mindfulness can assist control stress levels.

Education and Awareness: Increasing awareness about the impacts of sugar on health and advocating healthier alternatives might inspire better dietary choices. Educational initiatives and public health campaigns play a significant part in this effort.

Technology and Tools

Continuous Glucose Monitors (CGMs): For persons with diabetes, CGMs provide real-time data on blood glucose levels, helping to manage and prevent excessive changes.

Dental Technologies: Advances in dental technology, such as laser treatments and improved materials for fillings and crowns, enhance the effectiveness of dental care.

Balancing Act: How to Enjoy Sugar Without Harm

Enjoying sugar without compromising health demands a conscious and balanced approach. While sugar is typically demonized, it may be part of a healthy diet when ingested in moderation. The answer is in understanding how to balance sugar intake with other dietary and lifestyle choices.

Moderation and Portion Control

One of the most efficient methods to enjoy sugar without harm is by adopting moderation. This entails being cautious of portion amounts and the frequency of sugar consumption. For example, instead of eliminating sweets, you can enjoy smaller servings and limit them to occasional treats rather than regular indulgences.

Choosing Quality Over Quantity

Opt for high-quality, nutrient-dense foods that include natural sugars rather than manufactured ones with added sugars. Fruits, for example, supply natural sugars combined with necessary vitamins, minerals, and fiber. When you choose to consume sweets, picking those prepared with whole ingredients might offer a more enjoyable and healthier experience.

Reading Labels and Being Informed

Understanding food labels is vital for managing sugar intake. Many processed goods include hidden sugars under many labels, such as high fructose corn syrup, sucrose, glucose, and maltose. By reading labels and being aware of this varied terminology, you can make more educated decisions and avoid unneeded added sugars.

Incorporating Balanced Meals

Balancing meals with a variety of macronutrients—carbohydrates, proteins, and fats—helps manage blood sugar levels and decreases sugar cravings. For instance, pairing a sugary treat with a source of protein or healthy fat will limit the absorption of sugar into the bloodstream, reducing spikes and falls in blood sugar levels.

Mindful Eating Practices

Practicing mindful eating requires giving complete attention to the experience of eating, including the taste, texture, and perfume of food. This method encourages slower eating, which can lead to greater satisfaction with fewer portions and a better understanding of hunger and satiety cues. Mindful eating helps prevent overconsumption of sugary foods and fosters a healthier relationship with food.

Limiting Sugary Beverages

Sugary drinks, such as sodas, fruit juices, and sweetened teas, are a substantial source of added sugars in many diets. These beverages can contribute to abrupt rises in blood sugar levels and provide empty calories with little nutritious value. Replacing sugary drinks with water, herbal teas, or sparkling water with a splash of fruit juice will help reduce sugar intake.

Setting Realistic Goals

Setting reasonable targets for lowering sugar consumption might make the process more bearable.

Gradually cutting back on sugar, rather than making sudden changes, allows your taste buds to adjust and helps create durable habits. For example, if you regularly add two teaspoons of sugar to your coffee, try lowering it to one and eventually to none over time.

Healthy Alternatives and Substitutes

Exploring healthier alternatives to sugar can be useful. Natural sweeteners like honey, maple syrup, and stevia can deliver sweetness with fewer calories and added benefits. However, it's vital to utilize these alternatives in moderation, as they still include sugars or sugar-like substances.

Regular Physical Activity

Incorporating regular physical activity into your regimen helps balance blood sugar levels and maintain weight. Exercise improves insulin sensitivity, allowing your body to use glucose more effectively. Aim for a balance of cardio exercises, such as walking or cycling, and strength training to enhance health advantages.

Seeking Professional Guidance

For personalized guidance on managing sugar intake, engaging with healthcare professionals, such as dietitians or nutritionists, might be useful. They give specific advice based on your health state, dietary preferences, and lifestyle.

Psychological Effects: The Relationship Between Sugar and Mental Health

The relationship between sugar and mental health is nuanced and multifaceted. While sugar is typically connected with pleasure and reward, excessive consumption can have adverse consequences on mental well-being. Understanding these impacts can help individuals make informed choices regarding their sugar intake.

Short-Term Mood Boosts

Sugar consumption is known to produce a fast boost in mood and energy levels. This is due to the production of dopamine, a neurotransmitter associated with pleasure and reward, which occurs when we consume sweet meals. This temporary high can generate a sense of euphoria and fulfillment, which is why many individuals go for sweets in times of stress or emotional anguish.

The Cycle of Cravings and Energy Crashes

The short-term mood boost from sugar is generally followed by a quick drop in blood sugar levels, leading to energy dumps and irritation. This cycle of highs and lows might contribute to mood swings and increasing cravings for more sweets to recapture the initial sensation of pleasure. Over time, this can evolve into a dependence on sugar for emotional regulation, producing an unhealthy relationship with food.

Impact on Stress and Anxiety

While sugar can provide a momentary reprieve from stress, excessive consumption may aggravate stress and anxiety in the long run. High sugar intake has been related to elevated levels of cortisol, the body's major stress hormone. Elevated cortisol levels can disturb normal physiological activities and contribute to chronic stress and anxiety disorders.

Link to Depression

Emerging research reveals a potential link between high sugar consumption and depression. Diets heavy in added sugars and refined carbohydrates have been related to an increased risk of depression. This may be related to the inflammatory effects of sugar on the body and brain, as well as its impact on gut health, which plays a role in mood regulation.

Cognitive Function and Memory

Excessive sugar intake can also damage cognitive function and memory. Studies have demonstrated that diets rich in sugar can impair learning and memory by increasing inflammation in the brain and lowering the production of brain-derived neurotrophic factor (BDNF), a protein needed for brain function. This can lead to difficulty in concentration, decision-making, and overall cognitive performance.

Addictive Properties of Sugar

The concept of sugar addiction is a source of controversy among researchers. Some studies suggest that sugar can trigger the brain's reward circuits like addictive substances like drugs and alcohol. This activation can lead to increasing tolerance, where more sugar is needed to get the same pleasurable impact, and withdrawal symptoms when sugar intake is reduced.

Gut-Brain Axis

The gut-brain axis refers to as the bidirectional communication between the gut and the brain. A healthy gut microbiome has a significant role in mental health, impacting mood, anxiety, and cognitive processes. High-sugar diets can disturb the balance of good bacteria in the stomach, leading to dysbiosis, which has been related to mental health disorders such as depression and anxiety.

Strategies for Managing Sugar's Impact on Mental Health

Balanced Diet: Eating a balanced diet rich in whole foods, such as fruits, vegetables, whole grains, lean meats, and healthy fats, enhances mental health by supplying critical nutrients for brain function and lowering inflammation.

Mindfulness and Emotional Eating: Practicing mindfulness can help individuals become more aware of their eating behaviors and the emotional triggers that contribute to sugar cravings. Developing healthier coping methods for stress and emotions might lessen reliance on sugar for comfort.

Regular Exercise: Physical activity increases mood and decreases stress by increasing the synthesis of endorphins and promoting general well-being. Exercise also improves insulin sensitivity, which can help stabilize blood sugar levels.

Adequate Sleep: Ensuring sufficient and quality sleep is vital for mental health. Poor sleep can lead to increased desires for sweet foods and exacerbate mood issues. Establishing a regular sleep regimen can help alleviate these consequences.

Hydration: Staying hydrated is vital for general health and can help prevent sugar cravings. Sometimes, thirst is mistakenly for hunger, leading to unnecessary sugar consumption.

Help Systems: Seeking help from friends, family, or mental health experts can give the motivation and accountability needed to reduce sugar intake and improve mental health.

Chapter 8

Balancing Sugar in Your Diet

Balancing sugar in your diet entails making intentional choices about the types and amounts of sugar you consume. The goal is not to remove sugar totally but to ensure that it complements a good and varied diet. Start with being aware of your current sugar intake and identifying places where you may make adjustments.

Focus on consuming entire meals, such as fruits, vegetables, whole grains, lean proteins, and healthy fats, which give important nutrients and naturally occurring carbohydrates. These foods assist in maintaining stable blood sugar levels and provide sustained energy. Reserve additional sugars for special events and sweets, rather than making them a regular component of your diet.

Portion management is essential when it comes to managing sugar intake. Enjoying smaller servings of sugary foods can fulfill cravings without leading to overconsumption. For example, taste a small piece of dark chocolate instead of a full candy bar. Additionally, mixing sweet foods with fiber, protein, or fat can decrease the absorption of sugar into the bloodstream, minimizing the risk of blood sugar increases.

Another method is to minimize the quantity of sugar you add to foods and beverages. Gradually decreasing the quantity of sugar in your coffee, tea, or homemade foods allows your taste buds to adjust over time, making lower-sugar options more pleasant. Opt for natural sweetness from fruits or spices, such as cinnamon or vanilla, to improve flavor without relying on additional sugars.

Healthy Alternatives: Natural Sweeteners and Their Benefits

Natural sweeteners can be a healthier option to conventional sugars, giving sweetness with added nutritional advantages. These options include honey, maple syrup, agave nectar, coconut sugar, and stevia. While they should be used in moderation, natural sweeteners can deliver vitamins, minerals, and antioxidants that are absent in refined sugar.

Honey is a natural sweetener rich in antioxidants, vitamins, and minerals. It has antimicrobial effects and helps ease sore throats. However, it is still high in fructose and should be taken carefully, especially for persons controlling blood sugar levels.

Maple syrup is another natural sweetener that contains important antioxidants and minerals including manganese and zinc. It has a lower glycemic index than refined sugar, which means it has a reduced impact on blood sugar levels. Choose pure maple syrup over flavored syrups that contain extra sugars and artificial additives.

Agave nectar is made from agave plant. It has a low glycemic index but is heavy in fructose, which might have detrimental health effects if ingested in big amounts. Use agave nectar cautiously and be mindful of its fructose content.

Coconut sugar is manufactured from the sap of coconut palm plants and contains trace levels of vitamins and minerals. It has a lower glycemic index compared to refined sugar and preserves some of the nutrients contained in the coconut palm. Despite its benefits, coconut sugar should still be used in moderation.

Stevia is a natural, zero-calorie sweetener obtained from the leaves of the Stevia rebaudiana plant. It is substantially sweeter than sugar, thus only a small amount is needed to reach the appropriate level of sweetness. Stevia does not affect blood sugar levels, making it a viable alternative for persons with diabetes or those trying to reduce calorie intake. Ensure that you purchase pure stevia products without extra fillers or fake additives.

Reading Labels: Understanding Nutritional Labels to Make Informed Choices

Understanding nutritional labels is vital for making informed choices about the foods you consume, especially when it comes to regulating sugar intake. Nutritional labels contain information about the number of sugars, both natural and added, present in a food. By learning to read and interpret these labels, you may better regulate your sugar consumption and make healthier decisions.

Start by looking at the serving size and the quantity of servings per container. This information is significant because the sugar content mentioned on the label is based on the serving size. It consumes more than the recommended serving size means you'll be ingesting more sugar than indicated on the label.

Next, study the total carbs column, where sugars are stated. The label will differentiate between total sugars and added sugars. Total sugars comprise both natural sugars are (initiate in fruits, vegetables, and dairy products) and added sugars (those added during processing or preparation). Added sugars are a key health concern and should be restricted.

Common names for added sugars include sucrose, high fructose corn syrup, cane sugar, corn syrup, agave nectar, and honey. Familiarize yourself with these terms so you can recognize additional sugars in the ingredient list.

Understanding the percentage of daily value (%DV) it can help you understand how much sugar is in a product relative to a regular daily intake. The %DV for added sugars is based on a 2,000-calorie diet, with a recommendation to keep added sugars below 10% of total daily calories. This implies ingesting no more than 50 grams (12 teaspoons) of added sugars each day.

Be wary of items marketed as "low-fat" or "fat-free," as they often contain larger amounts of added sugars to compensate for the loss in fat. Similarly, goods advertised as "healthy" or "natural" might nonetheless contain considerable levels of added sugars. Always check the labels to make educated choices.

Mindful Consumption: Strategies for Reducing Sugar Intake Without Feeling Deprived

Reducing sugar intake doesn't have to mean feeling deprived. By adopting mindful consumption practices, you can enjoy your favorite foods while keeping a healthier diet. Mindful eating encourages you to pay attention to what and how you eat, developing a better relationship with food.

Start by identifying the sources of additional sugars in your diet. Common culprits include sugary beverages, snacks, desserts, and processed foods. Replace these with healthy alternatives. For example, switch sugary sodas for sparkling water with a splash of citrus or a few fresh berries. Choose entire fruits over fruit drinks or sweetened snacks to fulfill your sweet cravings healthily.

Plan your meals and snacks to include a balance of macronutrients—proteins, fats, and carbohydrates. This balance helps normalize blood sugar levels and lowers cravings for sugary foods. Incorporate high-fiber foods, such as whole grains, legumes, fruits, and vegetables, which give sustained energy and increase satiety.

Practicing portion control can dramatically alter your sugar intake. Serve smaller servings of desserts and sweets, and relish each bite. Eating slowly allows you to thoroughly savor the flavors and textures of your food, making you less inclined to overeat.

Create a supportive environment by keeping unhealthy, sugary snacks out of sight and equipping your kitchen with healthier options. Having healthy snacks readily available makes it easy to make healthier choices when hunger strikes.

Experiment with recipes to minimize the sugar content. Many recipes can be adapted to utilize less sugar without affecting taste. For instance, consider lowering the sugar in baked products by one-third to one-half and using natural sweeteners like applesauce, mashed bananas, or dates.

Stay hydrated, as thirst is sometimes misinterpreted as hunger or desire. Drinking plenty of water throughout the day can help lessen the craving for sugary snacks and beverages.

Finally, cultivate mindful enjoyment. When you do choose to have a sweet treat, enjoy it totally without guilt. Savor the event and acknowledge that it's a special occasion rather than a habit.

By using these tactics, you can limit your sugar intake while still enjoying the foods you love. Mindful consumption supports a balanced approach to eating, helping you maintain a nutritious diet without feeling deprived.

Healthy Alternatives: Natural Sweeteners and Their Pros/Cons

Natural sweeteners offer a means to reduce refined sugar intake while still enjoying sweetness in your diet. Each natural sweetener has its particular properties, benefits, and drawbacks, making them appropriate for varied needs and preferences.

Honey: Honey is a natural sweetener rich in antioxidants, vitamins, and minerals. It has antimicrobial effects and helps ease sore throats. Pros include its natural nature and nutritional benefits. Cons include its high calorie and fructose content, which might alter blood sugar levels if ingested in significant quantities. Honey should be used cautiously, especially for persons with diabetes or those seeking to maintain their weight.

Maple Syrup: Derived from the sap of maple trees, maple syrup includes important antioxidants and minerals including manganese and zinc. It has a lower glycemic index than refined sugar, which indicates it has a less substantial impact on blood sugar levels. The positives of maple syrup include its nutritional value and natural production procedure. The drawbacks are its high-calorie content and the potential for adulteration with added sugars, so it's crucial to purchase pure maple syrup.

Agave Nectar: Agave nectar is a sweetener obtained from the agave plant. It has a low glycemic index, making it a popular choice for folks wanting to prevent blood sugar spikes. However, it is high in fructose, which can have detrimental health effects if ingested in large amounts. The positives of agave nectar include its natural origin and low glycemic index. The negatives are its high fructose content and its impact on health issues like insulin resistance and fatty liver disease when ingested excessively.

Coconut Sugar: Made from the sap of coconut palm trees, coconut sugar maintains some minerals found in the coconut palm, such as iron, zinc, calcium, and potassium. It has a lower glycemic guide compared to refined sugar. Pros include its trace minerals and lower glycemic impact. Cons include its caloric content, similar to conventional sugar, and it should still be used in moderation.

Stevia: Stevia is a natural, zero-calorie sweetener obtained from the leaves of the Stevia rebaudiana plant. It is substantially sweeter than sugar, thus only a small amount is needed. Stevia does not affect blood sugar levels, making it suitable for those with diabetes or those lowering calorie intake. Pros include its zero-calorie composition and suitability for blood sugar management. Cons can include its aftertaste and possibly gastrointestinal discomfort in some persons when ingested in big amounts.

Cooking and Baking with Less Sugar

Cooking and baking with less sugar is a realistic technique to decrease overall sugar intake without compromising taste. By making clever tweaks, you can enjoy healthier versions of your favorite meals.

When baking, you can often cut the sugar level of a recipe by up to one-third without a major influence on texture or flavor. For instance, if a recipe calls for one cup of sugar, try using two-thirds of a cup instead. This modest adjustment can make a large difference in overall sugar consumption.

Natural sweeteners can be used as alternatives to refined sugar. For example, honey and maple syrup can replace sugar in many recipes, but you may need to modify the liquid level since these sweeteners add moisture. Typically, you should reduce the amount of other liquids in the recipe by roughly one-quarter for every cup of liquid sweetener used.

Spices and extracts are fantastic instruments for boosting flavor without adding sugar. Vanilla essence, almond extract, and spices like cinnamon, nutmeg, and cardamom can make baked goods taste sweeter without added sugar. Citrus zest from lemons, limes, and oranges can also offer a vibrant, sweet flavor

Recipes and Tips for Reducing Sugar in Home Cooking

Creating great dishes with less sugar involves easy swaps and inventive strategies. Here are some recipes and tips to help you get started:

Banana Oat Muffins: These muffins use ripe bananas to offer natural sweetness, avoiding the need for added sugar. Combine mashed bananas with oats, eggs, baking powder, and a splash of vanilla essence. Bake till golden brown for a healthy breakfast or snack choice.

Homemade Granola: Store-bought granola generally contains large levels of sugar. Make your own by mixing rolled oats with nuts, seeds, and a small quantity of honey or maple syrup. Bake till crispy, and serve with yogurt or milk.

Spaghetti Sauce: Many commercial pasta sauces have added sugars. Make your own by sautéing onions and garlic, then adding crushed tomatoes, herbs, and a sprinkle of salt. Let it simmer until thickened for a tasty, sugar-free sauce.

Smoothies: Instead of utilizing fruit juice as a foundation, opt for whole fruits and vegetables. Blend a combination of berries, spinach, Greek yogurt, and a splash of almond milk for a nutrient-dense smoothie with no additional sugar.

Salad Dressings: Commercial dressings might be heavy in sugar. Make your own by whisking together olive oil, vinegar, mustard, and herbs. For a touch of sweetness, add a small bit of honey or a splash of orange juice.

Flavor Enhancement Without Added Sugar

Enhancing the flavor of your dishes without added sugar entails using herbs, spices, and other natural ingredients to bring out the best in your food. These approaches can make your meals more pleasurable and help lessen your reliance on sugar.

Herbs & Spices: Fresh and dried herbs like basil, cilantro, mint, rosemary, thyme, and parsley give depth and richness to meals. Spices such as cinnamon, ginger, turmeric, and cloves can provide natural sweetness and warmth. Experiment with diverse combinations to find what you like best.

Acidic Ingredients: Ingredients like vinegar, citrus juice, and tomatoes can brighten flavors and minimize the need for added sugar. A dash of lemon or lime juice can boost the taste of a dish, making it brighter and more enjoyable.

Umami-high Foods: Food's high in umami, such as mushrooms, soy sauce, miso, and aged cheeses, can enhance savory flavors and diminish the craving for sweetness. Incorporating these elements into your cooking can provide depth and delight.

Natural Sweetness: Use naturally sweet veggies like carrots, sweet potatoes, and beets to add sweetness to your dishes. Roasting these vegetables caramelizes their natural sugars, boosting their sweetness without the need for added sugar.

Caramelization: Cooking techniques including roasting, grilling, and caramelizing can bring out the natural sweetness in foods. For example, roasting onions and bell peppers increases their sweetness, making them a tasty complement to salads, sandwiches, and main courses.

Fermented Foods: Fermented foods like sauerkraut, kimchi, and pickles contribute sour and nuanced flavors that can balance and enhance other ingredients. These foods also give probiotic advantages, helping to overall wellness.

Infused Water: Instead of sugary beverages, consider infusing water with fresh fruits, herbs, and spices. Combinations like cucumber and mint, lemon and ginger, or strawberry and basil deliver refreshing flavors without additional sugar.

By adding these strategies and products to your cooking, you can produce tasty, satisfying meals that are reduced in sugar. This method not only helps reduce overall sugar intake but also fosters a more diversified and tasty diet.

Chapter 9

The Food Industry and Sugar

The food industry has had a key impact on the prominence of sugar in our diets. From the early days of sugar cultivation and commerce to modern-day manufacturing, the industry's effect is extensive. The industry's principal purpose is to manufacture items that appeal to consumers, ensuring recurrent purchases. Sugar, being a very pleasant and cost-effective component, is a significant instrument in reaching this goal. It enhances flavor, texture, and shelf life, making it a favorite among food manufacturers. However, the increased use of sugar has important implications for public health, contributing to rising rates of obesity, diabetes, and other chronic illnesses.

Marketing Tactics: How the Food Industry Promotes Sugary Products

The food industry's marketing strategies are complex and smart, aimed to make sugary items appealing to a wide spectrum of consumers. These approaches frequently start with branding and packaging, which are created to draw attention and convey messages of health and happiness. Bright colors, entertaining characters, and enticing imagery are widely utilized to target children and their parents, generating an emotional connection that might impact purchasing decisions.

Advertising is another effective tool. Television advertising, online ads, and social media campaigns regularly promote the joyful experience of ingesting sweet food. They usually portray joyful, active people using the product, suggesting that it may offer joy and enhance one's lifestyle. Endorsements by celebrities and influencers further reinforce these ideas, giving a layer of credibility and aspirational appeal.

Promotional methods, including discounts, buy-one-get-one-free deals, and loyalty programs, entice consumers to purchase sugary items in bigger numbers. These campaigns are typically intentionally timed around holidays and special events when people are more prone to indulge.

Health claims might also be misleading. Terms like "low-fat," "natural," or "contains real fruit" can convey the idea that a product is healthier than it is, despite its high sugar content. This can persuade consumers to overlook the sugar content, feeling they are making a healthier option.

Hidden Sugars: Identifying Hidden Sugars in Processed Foods

Hidden sugars are a serious concern in processed foods. These sugars are introduced during manufacture and may not be instantly recognizable by customers. They often emerge under many identities, making it challenging to determine their presence.

Common names for added sugars include sucrose, high fructose corn syrup, agave nectar, maltose, dextrose, and others. Even products that don't taste unduly sweet, such as bread, salad dressings, and pasta sauces, can contain large amounts of hidden sugars.

Reading nutrition labels and ingredient lists is vital for discovering hidden sugars. The Nutrition Facts panel offers information on the total sugars in a product, which consist of both natural and added sugars. The ingredient list might show the precise types of sugars used, commonly presented in descending order by weight. Consumers should be mindful of phrases like "cane juice," "evaporated cane syrup," "fruit juice concentrates," and others that indicate additional sugars.

Understanding serving sizes is also vital. A product may appear low in sugar per serving, but if the serving size is excessively small, consumers may consume more sugar than intended.

Policy and Regulation: Government Actions to Control Sugar Consumption

Governments worldwide have acknowledged the public health dangers connected with increased sugar consumption and have developed numerous policies and legislation to address the issue. These measures attempt to minimize sugar intake, encourage healthier diets, and eventually enhance population health.

One popular technique is the imposition of sugar taxes. Several countries and towns have put tariffs on sugary beverages, which are often heavy in added sugars and drunk in big quantities. These levies are aimed at curbing consumption by increasing the cost of sugary drinks, so encouraging consumers to pick healthier alternatives. Studies have indicated that sugar tariffs might lead to a considerable decrease in the purchasing and consumption of sugary beverages.

Nutrition labeling requirements are another key instrument. Many nations require food manufacturers to explicitly identify the number of added sugars on product labels. This transparency helps consumers make informed decisions and motivates manufacturers to reformulate products with lower sugar content. In the United States, for example, the Food and Drug Administration (FDA) has ordered that added sugars be included on the Nutrition Facts panel, a law that came into full force in 2020.

Restrictions on advertising, particularly to youngsters, are also being implemented. The purpose is to restrict the exposure of youngsters to marketing for high-sugar foods and beverages. Countries like the United Kingdom have enacted restrictions that ban the advertising of unhealthy foods during children's television programming and on websites aimed at children.

Educational initiatives are vital for raising knowledge about the health effects of excessive sugar consumption and promoting healthier eating habits. Governments and public health organizations regularly launch these campaigns to provide information on how to minimize sugar intake and adopt healthier alternatives. These activities can include school-based programs, community workshops, and mass media campaigns.

Support for better food environments is another policy area. Governments can affect the availability of healthy food options through efforts such as giving subsidies for fruits and vegetables, promoting farmers' markets, and ensuring healthy foods are available in schools, workplaces, and public institutions. These initiatives make it easier for people to access and choose healthy options over sugary ones.

The food industry has played a big part in pushing and embedding sugar into our daily diets through creative marketing, hidden sugars in processed goods, and extensive use of health claims. Government initiatives, including sugar levies, labeling requirements, advertising limitations, educational programs, and support for better food environments, are vital in tackling the public health concern caused by excessive sugar intake.

By understanding these dynamics, consumers may make more educated choices and fight for legislation that favors healthy dietary patterns.

Chapter 10

Moving Forward

As we look ahead, the task of limiting sugar consumption becomes increasingly crucial. With rising rates of obesity, diabetes, and other chronic diseases associated with high sugar intake, there is a clear need for continuous initiatives to encourage healthier eating habits. Moving forward requires a multi-faceted approach, encompassing public health programs, individual efforts, and innovations in food production and consumption.

Public Health Initiatives: Successful Programs and Initiatives to Reduce Sugar Consumption

Public health programs play a key role in lowering sugar intake on a large basis. Several successful programs have proven the benefit of coordinated efforts to promote healthier eating.

One famous example is the "Sugar Smart" campaign in the United Kingdom, developed by Public Health England. This project attempted to educate the public about the consequences of excessive sugar intake and provided practical recommendations on how to limit sugar consumption. The campaign included a smartphone app that allowed users to scan barcodes of food goods to determine their sugar level, making it easier for consumers to make informed choices. Additionally, the program worked with schools to enhance the nutritional content of meals and teach youngsters about healthy eating.

In Mexico, a sugar tax on sugary beverages has proven favorable outcomes. Introduced in 2014, the tax resulted in a considerable decline in the purchasing of sugary drinks, particularly among low-income households. Revenue from the levy has been utilized to pay for public health activities, including the installation of water fountains in schools, further encouraging healthy alternatives to sugary beverages.

The United States has also had effective efforts, such as the Healthy Food Financing Initiative (HFFI). This initiative aims to enhance access to healthy foods in marginalized communities by encouraging the construction of grocery stores, farmers' markets, and other food retail outlets. By boosting the availability of healthy food options, the HFFI helps minimize dependency on processed meals high in added sugars.

Personal Stories: Case Studies of Individuals Who Have Reduced Their Sugar Intake

Personal tales and case studies give strong evidence of the benefits of lowering sugar intake. These narratives can motivate others to make similar changes and highlight practical techniques for cutting back on sugar.

One such story is that of Jane, a mother of two who resolved to minimize her family's sugar consumption after her children were diagnosed with prediabetes. Jane began by reading labels more carefully and eliminating unhealthy foods and drinks from her household. She brought more fruits, vegetables, and whole grains into their diet, and discovered inventive ways to make meals pleasurable without added sweeteners. Over time, her children's health improved, and their prediabetes was reversed. Jane's tale underlines the importance of parental influence and proactive dietary modifications.

Another case is that of Mark, a middle-aged guy who struggled with obesity and high blood pressure. After attending a community health session, he learned about the influence of sugar on his health and decided to take action. Mark started by cutting out sugary beverages and decreasing his intake of processed foods. He replaced them with water, herbal teas, and cooked meals. As a result, Mark lost significant weight, his blood pressure corrected, and he reported feeling more energized and focused.

These personal stories show the transforming power of lowering sugar intake. They illustrate that with determination and assistance, individuals can make major health changes.

Future Trends: Innovations and Future Directions in Managing Sugar Consumption

Looking to the future, various trends and breakthroughs promise to further promote the reduction of sugar consumption. Advances in food technology, regulatory changes, and alterations in consumer behavior are all leading to a healthier food landscape.

One interesting trend is the development of novel sweeteners that deliver the flavor of sugar without the calories. Natural sweeteners like stevia and monk fruit extract have gained popularity as alternatives to regular sugar. Additionally, scientists are focusing on generating synthetic sweeteners that match the taste and functional features of sugar while being digested differently by the body, potentially minimizing health hazards.

Another innovation is the reformulation of food products by manufacturers. In response to consumer demand and governmental pressure, many companies are decreasing the sugar level in their products. This involves employing alternative sweeteners, increasing natural tastes, and improving the overall nutritional profile of foods. Reformulated goods allow consumers to enjoy familiar foods with less sugar, making healthier choices easier.

Policy changes continue to play a key effect. Governments around the world are establishing stronger rules on sugar content, labeling, and marketing. These regulations help create an environment where healthy choices are more accessible and desirable. For example, mandated front-of-package labeling systems that highlight high sugar content can drive consumers toward healthier options.

Consumer behavior is also developing. Increasing knowledge of the health concerns linked with high sugar intake is increasing demand for healthier alternatives. People are becoming more attentive to their nutritional choices, seeking out whole foods, and preferring nutrition above convenience. This trend is motivating the food sector to innovate and deliver better options.

In addition to technological and policy breakthroughs, community-based methods are gaining appeal. Local efforts that encourage healthy eating, such as community gardens, cooking courses, and nutrition education programs, empower individuals to take responsibility for their meals. These programs frequently focus on underprivileged groups, addressing gaps in access to healthful meals.

Finally, the role of digital technology in regulating sugar consumption cannot be disregarded. Apps and online platforms that analyze food intake, provide individualized nutrition recommendations and offer support communities are becoming helpful tools for individuals wanting to reduce sugar intake. These technologies make it easier for people to assess their progress, set objectives, and stay motivated.

The future of managing sugar consumption seems optimistic, with a combination of novel sweeteners, food reformulation, regulatory reforms, altering consumer behavior, community initiatives, and digital technologies all contributing to a better diet. By being informed and making deliberate decisions, individuals may navigate the modern food scene and enjoy the benefits of lower sugar consumption.

Chapter 11

Recommendations and Guidelines

Understanding the recommendations and limits for sugar consumption is crucial for making informed nutritional choices. Health organizations worldwide provide guidelines to help individuals manage their sugar intake and preserve optimal health. The recommendations are based on substantial research and aim to lower the risk of chronic diseases related to high sugar consumption.

Expert Guidelines for Sugar Consumption (WHO, AHA, etc.)

Several health organizations have produced advice on sugar intake, including the World Health Organization (WHO) and the American Heart Association (AHA). These guidelines offer a framework for consumers to understand how much sugar is safe to consume and the potential health advantages of lowering sugar intake.

World Health Organization (WHO)

The WHO recommends that adults and children decrease their intake of free sugars to less than 10% of their total calorie intake. Free sugars contain monosaccharides and disaccharides added to foods and drinks, as well as sugars naturally present in honey, syrups, fruit juices, and fruit juice concentrates. For further health benefits, the WHO recommended decreasing the intake of free sugars to below 5% of total caloric intake. This translates to around 25 grams (around 6 teaspoons) of sugar per day for an average adult.

American Heart Association (AHA)

The AHA provides more detailed recommendations based on gender and age. It proposes that women limit their intake of added sugars to no more than 100 calories per day (about 6 teaspoons or 24 grams), while men should consume not more than 150 calories daily (about 9 teaspoons or 36 grams). For children, the AHA recommends that added sugars make up fewer than 25 grams (6 teaspoons) per day and discourages the intake of sugar-sweetened beverages for children under the age of 2.

Dietary Guidelines for Americans

The Dietary Guidelines for Americans, updated every five years from the U.S. Department of Health and Human Services and the U.S. Department of Agriculture, say that added sugars should make up less than 10% of daily calories. This guideline agrees with those of the WHO and highlights the need for nutrient-dense diets and beverages.

Individual Needs and Considerations

While broad guidelines are helpful, individual needs and factors must be taken into account when choosing an optimal level of sugar consumption. Factors such as age, gender, exercise level, overall diet, and health status can determine how much sugar an individual should ingest.

Age and Gender

Children and adolescents have distinct nutritional demands compared to adults. Growing bodies require appropriate energy and minerals, but it is crucial to balance this with avoiding added sweets to prevent obesity and dental concerns. Older folks may have other issues, such as treating chronic diseases like diabetes or heart disease, which demands careful control of sugar intake.

Activity Level

Physical exercise plays a crucial role in influencing energy demands and sugar intake. Active persons or athletes may require extra carbs, especially sugars, to fuel their performance and recovery. However, it is still vital to prioritize complex carbs and natural sources of sugar, such as fruits, over-processed and sugary foods.

Overall Diet

The quality of an individual's total diet should be addressed when measuring sugar intake. A diet high in nutrient-dense foods, such as vegetables, fruits, whole grains, lean proteins, and healthy fats, can provide some freedom in sugar consumption. Conversely, a diet high in processed foods and poor in vital nutrients may demand tougher limits on added sugars to maintain proper nutrition.

Health Status

Existing health issues, such as diabetes, obesity, and cardiovascular disease, necessitate special dietary changes. Individuals with diabetes need to check their blood sugar levels and control carbohydrate intake carefully. Those with obesity or heart disease may benefit from limiting added sugars to help manage weight and enhance cardiovascular health.

Personal Preferences and Lifestyle

Personal tastes and lifestyle choices also affect sugar consumption. Some individuals may find it simpler to adhere to a diet with minimal added sugars, while others may choose to incorporate occasional treats in moderation. Finding a sustainable balance that matches personal tastes might help preserve long-term adherence to healthy eating habits.

Cultural and Social Factors

Cultural and socioeconomic variables influence eating habits and sugar consumption patterns. Traditional diets and cultural traditions may involve the usage of particular sweeteners or sugary foods. It is crucial to honor cultural rituals while urging moderation and healthier alternatives where possible.

Strategies for Managing Sugar Intake

Understanding the standards is the first step, but practical solutions are important to limit sugar intake properly. Here are several techniques to assist individuals to minimize their sugar consumption while still enjoying their food:

1. Educate Yourself

Knowledge is power when it comes to managing sugar intake. Learning to read and comprehend nutrition labels can assist uncover hidden sugars in processed foods.

Look for components like high fructose corn syrup, sucrose, glucose, and other sweets.

2. Choose Whole Foods

Emphasizing whole, unadulterated foods might naturally lower sugar intake. Fruits, vegetables, whole grains, lean proteins, and healthy fats give necessary nutrients without the added sugars found in many processed diets.

3. Limit Sugary Beverages

Sugary drinks, such as soda, fruit juices, and energy drinks, are substantial sources of added sugars. Opt for water, unsweetened teas, or liquids sweetened with natural alternatives like stevia.

4. Be Mindful of Portion Sizes

Even when consuming sweet meals, being conscious of portion sizes can help limit overall sugar intake. Enjoying smaller portions of desserts and sweets might fulfill cravings without overindulging.

5. Plan and Prepare Meals

Preparing meals at home offers users' greater control over ingredients and sugar levels. Experimenting with recipes that use natural sweeteners or lowering the quantity of sugar in typical dishes can make a major difference.

6. Balance Macronutrients

Including a balance of carbohydrates, proteins, and fats in meals will help regulate blood sugar levels and prevent cravings for sugary snacks. Protein and healthy fats, in particular, can enhance satiety and lessen the urge for sweets.

7. Stay Active

Regular physical activity helps manage blood sugar levels and can reduce some of the detrimental consequences of sugar consumption. Exercise also helps overall health and well-being, making it simpler to maintain a balanced diet.

8. Seek Support

For people attempting to limit sugar intake, obtaining advice from healthcare professionals, dietitians, or support groups can provide guidance and encouragement. Personalized counsel and accountability can make the process more doable.

Navigating the world of sugar consumption demands a balance of recognizing professional advice and customizing it to individual requirements. By adopting practical tactics and making informed decisions, individuals can enjoy sugar in moderation while prioritizing their overall health and well-being.

Conclusion

In comprehending sugar and its impact on health, it is crucial to recognize the balance between enjoyment and moderation. This balance can help prevent potential health hazards linked with excessive sugar consumption while allowing for the odd indulgence.

Recap: Summarize the Key Points Discussed in the Book

This book has presented a full review of sugar, beginning with its definition and types, including natural sugars like sucrose, fructose, and glucose, as well as added sugars found in many processed foods. The history of sugar, from its ancient roots to its function in modern diets, was explored, showing its cultural relevance and economic impact.

The book discussed the manufacturing process of table sugar, the nutritional value it delivers, and the chemicals involved in its creation. Various myths and misconceptions regarding sugar were disproved, including the belief that Americans consume more sugar than ever, that sugar is innately addictive, and that white sugar is bleached.

The health implications of sugar consumption were thoroughly researched, revealing both short-term effects, such as blood glucose spikes, and long-term ramifications, including the increased risk of chronic diseases including obesity, diabetes, and heart disease. The book also examined the psychological impacts of sugar, emphasizing its impact on mental health and the possibility of cravings induced by dopamine responses.

Guidelines from renowned health organizations including the WHO and AHA were presented to provide a foundation for safe sugar consumption. Individual demands and considerations were underlined, underlining the significance of tailoring dietary choices based on criteria such as age, exercise level, overall diet, and health status.

Practical solutions for limiting sugar intake were presented, including recommendations for reading labels, choosing healthy alternatives, and implementing mindful consumption habits. The role of the food business and government restrictions in creating sugar consumption patterns was explored, providing insight into the broader context of dietary habits.

Final Thoughts: Encouragement and Motivation for Readers to Take Control of Their Sugar Consumption

Taking control of sugar consumption is a vital step toward reaching better health and well-being. While sugar can be part of a balanced diet, recognizing its effects and making informed decisions can greatly improve long-term health outcomes.

It is empowering to realize that little, incremental changes can lead to huge rewards. Reducing sugary beverages, choosing whole meals, and being conscious of portion sizes are all doable changes that can make a major difference. Remember, it's not about eliminating sugar but finding a balance that supports overall health without feeling deprived.

Support and resources are available for individuals wishing to make these changes. Healthcare professionals, nutritionists, and community initiatives can offer guidance and support. Personal tales and case studies of persons who have successfully reduced their sugar intake might serve as inspiration and encouragement.

Future trends in regulating sugar consumption look positive, with advancements in natural sweeteners and an increasing emphasis on public health programs. Staying updated about these developments might help folks make better decisions and adjust to new recommendations as they emerge.

By taking control of sugar consumption, individuals can optimize their health, prevent chronic diseases, and have a more balanced and meaningful lifestyle. The journey toward better behaviors is a constant process, but with the correct knowledge and tools, it is attainable.

* 9 7 9 8 3 3 5 3 8 1 6 8 0 *